HOW TO INITIATE YOUR OWN RED PILL REBELLION AND WIN

ESCAPE THE MEDICAL MATRIX

DR. VIC NAUMOV

Disclaimer:
Consult a medical doctor or other licensed medical professional if you suffer from any medical conditions. This publication presents only the author's opinions, which are based on his knowledge, experiences and beliefs. This book and its contents do not cure, prevent, diagnose or treat any disease or condition. The purpose of this book is educational, research and entertainment. The information contained within this book is for informational purposes only. The author, the publisher and everybody involved with the publication, distribution or sale of this book assume no responsibility.

CONTENTS

DEDICATION 4

PREFACE 5

INTRODUCTION 7

CHAPTER 1:

WELCOME TO THE REBELLION: YOUR RED PILL OFFER 9

CHAPTER 2:

THE ARCHITECT: OVERLORDS & BLUEPRINT
OF THE MEDICAL MATRIX 13

CHAPTER 3:

1969: EVIDENCE OF A SECRET MEDICAL SEMINAR
TASKED TO TRANSFORM AMERICA 31

CHAPTER 4:

THE SYSTEM ENGAGED: THEIR GREAT RESET AGENDA 65

CHAPTER 5:

YOUR MORPHEUS MOMENT: THE SIMULATION
FURTHER EXPOSED 97

CHAPTER 6:

THE ORACLE: KNOW THYSELF & THE SACRED SECRET ... 135

CHAPTER 7:

YOU ARE THE ONE: IT HAS ALWAYS BEEN ABOUT YOU! 141

ABOUT THE AUTHOR 148

DEDICATION

To my beautiful, loving and amazing wife of over thirty years, Colleen. You have and always will be my ride or die. To my two amazing sons, Bryant and Conor, I exposed and fought through the lies of the Medical Matrix so both of you could grow up healthy, vibrant and strong outside of it. I hope everything I taught you will pass down to your future children because only health is true wealth. Finally, to all the brave mothers and fathers continuing to fight daily for medical freedom. You are not alone and must understand the fact that, "Freedom isn't free. It requires rebellion." I salute you!

PREFACE

"You're here because you know something. What you know you can't explain, but you feel it. You've felt it your entire life, that there's something wrong with the world. You don't know what it is, but it's there, like a splinter in your mind, driving you mad."

– Morpheus speaking to Neo from *The Matrix* movie

In a sick society, prioritizing one's health becomes the ultimate form of rebellion. You must understand, you were born into the "Medical Matrix" against your will; an artificial simulation designed to create the illusion of producing health, vitality and longevity, but in reality creates sickness, suffering and lifelong dependency on it. It is an integrated system of lies and control created to be a virus of the mind, implanted in each child and then continues to grow, replicate and manifest into adulthood and continues throughout life. Since 1913 there has been no cure, until now.

Under natural law, you were born to be healthy, but within the Medical Matrix you were raised to be sick. Health is humanity's natural state. The time is now, to reclaim it and escape the Medical Matrix for good.

The power of choice is now yours. This book is written for those who are awake, ready to get off their knees and are prepared to end the virus of the mind that has enslaved them. Get ready to initiate your own "Red Pill Rebellion" and WIN.

INTRODUCTION

"Since 1913, we Americans have been living in a simulated Medical Matrix, deliberately divided into two distinct sects, those with power and those without. Welcome to the rebellion. I don't know the future. I didn't write this book to tell you how this is going to end. I wrote this book to tell you how it was going to begin."

– Dr. Vic Naumov, DC

Our health, vitality and longevity are controlled by an artificial simulation that I have termed the "Medical Matrix," whose Architect in the United States of America was House of Rothschild agent John D. Rockefeller Sr., who launched the Medical Matrix in 1913. Most everything you have been programmed to believe in and trust is nothing but an illusion to keep you trapped in the health care/sickness system of control. Our physical, chemical and mental worlds are primarily run by the Rockefeller Foundation and the World Health Organization (WHO), both of which are designed to profit off of your pain and suffering. Fear and ignorance are their two avenues of manipulation. They use media outlets, celebrities, movies, engineered foods and mind manipulation tactics to keep the people enslaved within a system that doesn't serve them. In order to regain health, vitality and freedom, we must dismantle the Medical Matrix to prevent the "Great Reset." To do this, we must stop being their customers, and understand that each of us possesses the innate power to heal from within and need to rediscover how to nurture nature. We must raise the human consciousness and cleanse the lower vibrational feelings of fear, shame and guilt. Collectively, in letting go of our fear, we cannot be controlled, manipulated or destroyed. We must stand together in our innate truth, understanding and light; only then will we escape the control of the Rockefeller Foundation's Medical Matrix or fall victim to the global Great Reset. As a result, we will finally be able to get out of "Generation SICK" and restore freedom, liberty and self-responsibility, just as our Creator intended.

CHAPTER 1

WELCOME TO THE REBELLION: YOUR RED PILL OFFER

"This is your last chance, after this, there is no turning back. You take the blue pill—the story ends, you wake up in your bed and believe whatever you want to believe. You take the red pill—you stay in wonderland and I show you how deep the rabbit hole goes."

– Morpheus speaking to Neo from *The Matrix* movie

Back in 2016, I wrote and published the groundbreaking book *Generation SICK*. This was my first attempt at pulling back the curtain of the "Medical Matrix" created by John D. Rockefeller Sr.

I chose the term Medical Matrix to describe the false reality Rockefeller created back in 1913 when he, along with his crony Abraham Flexner (i.e., the *Flexner Report*), deliberately hijacked and destroyed the naturally based American health care system. After its complete destruction and overhaul, the Rockefeller Foundation was created to sustain its dominance, impose its will and maintain its superiority. The nefarious scheme of the Rockefeller Foundation was to discredit, dismantle and disassociate humanity from all things natural. The foundation initiated the "Great Reset" for all educational and medical institutions in America. Which ultimately resulted in future generations not being able to learn, apply or understand the natural cosmic arrangement between man and his Creator. This false reality facilitated what we now understand is the Medical Matrix.

Since 1913, the Rockefeller Foundation has controlled every aspect of medicine, its educational schools and the practice of their doctors. To ensure the continued compliance of the American public, the foundation's propaganda, brainwashing tactics and indoctrination process have been forced upon each new generation. As a result, the Medical Matrix scheme has been implanted in the minds of every American man, woman and child. As a result, subconsciously people began to follow in blind faith and trust practices whenever they participated in the newly created "allopathic Rockefeller medical system."

Those who were plugged into the system were indoctrinated to view medical doctors as saviors and began worshiping at the altar of the white coat and never recognizing the fact that the Medical Matrix was created to enslave them physically, chemically and mentally. Keeping them and their loved ones in a constant cycle of sickness, all the while profiting off of their pain and suffering.

The Medical Matrix has such a deep and profound imprint on the subconscious mind of the American people that within just two generations the Rockefeller psyops was complete where toxic drugs, radical surgeries and long-term hospital stays had become the normal and accepted model of health care for all Americans. Without question or resistance, by virtue of blind faith, the previous model of health care that focused on nurturing nature was quickly replaced. As a result, the American people went from being one of the healthiest countries in the world to the sickest, yet this is not by accident, but by specific and calculated design. Thus paving the way for "Generation SICK," which still holds a firm grasp on American society, even today in 2024.

"Trust the science," "safe and effective," "two weeks to flatten the curve," "wear a mask," "stay six feet apart," "take the shot so you don't give or spread COVID," sound familiar? The year 2020 was a very interesting year, wasn't it? It launched a version of the Medical Matrix the world has never seen before. Those who were committed disciples complied and bent the knee without question to their master. The rest, questioned everything, believed nothing and did their own research. Now it's 2024 and the results are in. So, who made out better? Those who chose to take the blue pill, the disciples of the Medical Matrix or those who chose to take the red pill, the rebellious "Pure Bloods."

The lesson to be learned is never trust a system designed to keep you on your knees like a slave and profit off of your pain and suffering. It is important to understand these two factual statements: "There is no power without compliance" and "Freedom isn't free. It requires rebellion." The world was tested in 2020, some passed and others failed, but it was the Medical Matrix that won.

After the COVID "corona" pandemic was deliberately launched, the Rockefeller Foundation sprang into action. The psyops of fear, ignorance and the illusion of power quickly spread and many chose to comply with their tyrannical tactics. This was done all in the name of "public health." Now, four years removed from the global shutdown event, we can clearly see the aftermath. The Great Reset is upon us.

Some may think this was the first Medical Matrix attempt to "reset" American culture and bring the people to their knees, but it's not. In this book I will expose the first collective attempt to set forth a "Great American Reset" that was initiated and slowly implemented without your knowledge back in 1969. A secret medical seminar held back then where selected medical doctors (pediatricians specifically) were invited to participate and lay a new social foundational blueprint for the future. The purpose was to secretly and quietly transform America from within using pediatricians to serve as a parents' gateway medical doctor responsible for the children to enter the system.

The complete details of the secret seminar will be exposed within these pages giving you the knowledge and understanding of its plot, purpose and application. My intention for this book is to offer you the "red pill" to help you recognize and break free from the Medical Matrix and reject the Great Reset. In doing so we can finally regain our health, freedom and liberty while helping to once again, restore the "power to the people" where it ultimately belongs. The time to rise, get informed and take action is now! We all deserve the God-given opportunity to be happy, healthy and free!

CHAPTER 2

THE ARCHITECT: OVERLORDS & BLUEPRINT OF THE MEDICAL MATRIX

"Denial is the most predictable of all human responses."

– The Architect from *The Matrix* movie

The Hippocratic Oath serves as a reminder to medical doctors of their purpose and duty as health care professionals, but the practices of the medical profession today have little to do with the teachings and practices of Hippocrates. Hippocrates was a "naturopathic" physician who used natural techniques and natural substances such as herbs to treat and cure disease. Most doctors today have been trained, more so indoctrinated, into a system we can call "allopathic" medicine, which promotes the widespread use of artificial, chemically based drugs and surgical treatments rather than relying on the wisdom of the body to right itself when confronted by disease. The name and image of Hippocrates have been used as a smokescreen to hide the real purpose of modern medicine men and their allopathic system of medical care.

Throughout the last century, it is certainly true that major strides have been made in improving longevity and public health. While this progress is undeniable, the cause of this improvement is a matter of some controversy. While some surgical techniques and wonder drugs such as penicillin have justly made their inventors and discoverers known as benefactors of humanity, it has also been noted that much of the improvement in our quality and quantity of life comes from measures such as improving the drinking water supply, better diet and exercise habits, smoking cessation and reducing air pollution. For all the money our society spends on painkillers, sexual stimulants, blood thinners, and so on, drugs have had relatively little impact on the state of public health. Many of their benefits are sidelined by potent side effects, chemicals now poisoning our water supply, and by the decreasing effectiveness of drugs that have been way overprescribed (resistance to antibiotics is just one of the better-known examples).

Naturopathic doctors understand that human beings, as part of nature, are best treated with remedies that are natural. Fresh air, sunlight, clean water, healthy non-GMO food, herbal remedies, chiropractic, massage, acupuncture and positive thinking will do more to keep a person healthy and well balanced than a whole pharmacy full of pills, topical solutions and test kits. This does not mean that medical information is irrelevant or that all scientific progress in medicine is useless. On the contrary, the best naturopathic physicians are careful students of the body and its reactions to the environment.

They spend time getting to know their patients and building relationships with them based on the shared goal of promoting and living a healthy lifestyle. The main purpose of health care under this system is preventive medicine, that is, keeping a person from getting so sick that he or she ends up in the hospital or forms a lifelong dependence on powerful drugs. More and more, mainstream physicians recognize that the best advice a doctor can give is to encourage patients to eat properly, to exercise regularly, and to avoid introducing unnatural and harmful substances into the body.

The Rockefeller allopathic model of medicine, the Medical Matrix, was introduced to the United States not as a health care system, but rather as an industrial enterprise carefully designed and engineered to provide a steady stream of profit to the great monopolists of America's Gilded Age. America's current medical training system was pioneered largely in Germany, which had long been recognized as a leader in the fields of chemistry, pharmacology, medical use of radiation, surgery and hospital-building. This German model relied heavily on the use of drugs, surgical procedures and long hospital stays. It has gotten to the point that many Americans feel that a visit to the doctor has been wasted unless the patient is sent home with a pill prescription, a recommendation for a colonoscopy or a referral to an in-network specialist, who will offer an entirely new menu of potent and very expensive tests and treatments.

The Medical Matrix, that is, allopathic medicine, which means the shepherding of patients to ever more expensive surgical interventions and drug therapies, is purely profit-driven. Hospitals and drug research labs are mammoth enterprises that depend on the influx of a constantly increasing supply of patient money, whether generated through greater numbers of sick people or through higher charges for procedures. Considering, the generation of profits is the main priority of the health care system, healing and curing the sick becomes an afterthought. It is often noted that the vast majority of hospital care the average American receives over a lifetime occurs in the last year of their life. The longer an individual is kept sick and in a state of symptom management, the more money is generated to support the growth and expansion of the medical system.

Patients come to doctors hoping for cures; what they receive instead are "treatments," drugs or surgical procedures that at times are quite effective, but all too often only serve to exacerbate or prolong the condition that sent the patient to the doctor's office in the first place. That is because curing advocates actual healing and that goes directly against the Rockefeller Foundation's "allopathic medical" business model of creating customers, not cures.

The late Queen Elizabeth of England was probably the best-known advocate of homeopathy. Her personal physician, Dr. Peter Fisher, is a homeopath. He also treats other members of the royal family, including King Charles III. In the United States, homeopathic physicians are viewed as "quacks." The medical cartel makes attempts at every turn to discredit their work in the public square, but it was not so long ago that homeopathy was considered a mainstream approach that delivered good results for many patients.

Dr. George H. Simmons, who ran the American Medical Association from 1899–1924, for many years ran advertisements in Lincoln, Nebraska, where he practiced, which proudly proclaimed that he was a "homeopathic physician."

Homeopaths claimed notable success in treating major cholera epidemics in Europe, beginning with an 1831 epidemic that ravaged Europe. Patients treated in conventional hospitals suffered mortality rates from 40 percent to as high as 80 percent, while patients treated by homeopaths had a significantly lower death rate. In Bavaria, it was reported, only 7 percent of homeopathic patients died! The London Homeopathic Hospital claimed a 16.4 percent mortality rate during an 1854 outbreak that killed 51.8 percent of those treated allopathically.

Dr. Hahnemann's book *Homeopathica Materia Medica* made learning the art and methods of homeopathy quick and easy. As a result, in the nineteenth century, homeopathy expanded quite rapidly throughout the United States and Europe. It was so popular at the height of its success that homeopathic physicians outnumbered allopathic physicians by more than two to one.

In response to the rise in popularity of the homeopathic physicians, the American Medical Association (AMA) was founded as a trade lobby, for the purpose of neutralizing any competition and driving the homeopaths out of business.

By the early 1900s, the AMA was able, in large measure, to achieve these objectives.

The AMA not only attacked the homeopathic physicians, but also attacked any practitioner who practiced any form of healing that addresses the human body as a whole, rather than taking up one part at a time. Since allopathic physicians were trained to treat symptoms and not causes of disease, every practitioner who treated causes was seen as a threat, and was thereby exposed to attacks by the AMA.

The dogmas that fueled the illusion of the superiority of the AMA-run schools of medicine could be seen clearly in the constant self-promotion of their lies that the allopathic brand of medicine was the only type that was effective in the treatment of disease. This power-driven falsehood was responsible for creating the "godlike" egoistic ethos of the allopathic physician. This dangerous phenomenon of the supposed omniscient physician ("I know it all. Don't question me. I don't make mistakes.") lives on today in undiminished form, although it is increasingly under attack from nurse practitioners and patient advocates who favor a more patient-centered approach.

Ivan Illich, in his 1976 book *Medical Nemesis: the Expropriation of Health*, points out that the vaunted effectiveness of the allopathic school of medicine proved to be pure mythology and propaganda. Not only did doctors fail to stem the rising tide of chronic disease, even more disastrously, allopathic doctors brought new plagues into being, illnesses that Illich defines as "iatrogenic." He defines iatrogenic disease as an "illness which is caused by a doctor's medical intervention." Illich goes on to define three commonly encountered types of iatrogenesis: clinical iatrogenesis, which he defines as a doctor-made illness; social iatrogenesis, which is deliberately created by the mechanization of the medical-industrial complex; and cultural iatrogenesis, which he states, saps the people's will to survive.

Illich claims that this iatrogenesis plague is now sweeping the nation. One in twenty-five hospital patients nationwide acquire hospital-borne infections during their treatment. The problem is particularly acute in people who have to endure long-term stays. The rate of medical mistakes is so high that malpractice rates in some specialties are prohibitively expensive.

Dr. Atul Gawande, a leading surgeon who has written critically of his profession, has called for the adoption of a "checklist" system to ensure that fewer patients discover in the recovery room that the wrong lung has been removed, or that the wrong leg was amputated.

The Medical Matrix ensures we are indoctrinated from childhood with the idea that we should blindly trust medical doctors. Yet, how can this trust survive when, all too often, the professional who supposedly has been trained to heal you has been exposed as the same person who is now responsible for making you sick?

In its strive for power and control over the citizens of the United States, the AMA continues to push its claims that medical care has improved, and that it is largely as a result of their efforts that the health and longevity of the American citizens has also improved. Historical records show otherwise and debunk many of these claims. There is an abundance of evidence to support the idea that due to allopathic medical intervention, the health of the American people has declined in many respects. Any advances that did occur were often in spite of the doctors when mortality rates declined! Ignaz Semmelweis fought a losing battle in trying to get doctors to wash and disinfect their hands prior to treating patients in maternity wards. Even after he showed that deaths from "childbed fever" declined from 35 percent to as little as 1 percent among doctors taking this simple precaution. He failed to explain why it should be done, resulting in his work being mostly ignored. He was derided as a crank and never lived to see the adoption of hand washing just years after his untimely death, which occurred shortly after he was committed to an asylum.

Some argue that mortality rates from infectious diseases such as tuberculosis (TB) began their steep declines long before the introduction of vaccines and antibiotics. Late in the nineteenth century, it is estimated that 80 percent or more of the urban population in Europe and the United States was infected with the TB bacillus. Developing active TB was a death sentence: 80 percent of patients died from the disease. Poor sanitation and high population density contributed greatly to the spread of TB. As conditions improved due to the introduction of public health measures such as the introduction of running water and indoor plumbing to homes, the discouragement of spitting in the streets, and isolation of TB patients from the general population, rates began to fall. Thanks in large measure to the pioneering work of Robert

Koch and the development of antibiotics, TB has been nearly eliminated in the United States.

The effectiveness of antibiotics in the fight against TB has been proclaimed one of medical history's greatest success stories, but a balanced look at the history of TB treatment reveals that this is not a case of either/or. Homeopathic doctors dominated the American landscape in the nineteenth century, and as we have seen, the medical community, working with public health authorities, had already made considerable headway in reducing the toll from TB long before Koch succeeded in identifying its cause. Increasingly, we face the threat of drug-resistant strains of TB. In 2014, the National Institutes of Health (NIH) released a report on a study in India, where it was found that homeopathic treatment appeared to have some effectiveness when drugs were not working. The conclusion of the NIH report was that the use of homeopathy as an adjunct to traditional drug therapy merits further study.

The story with other infectious diseases, from whooping cough and diphtheria to polio, is much the same. Despite all the progress medical science has made since Pasteur and Koch established the germ theory of disease, we are still groping for effective treatments for cancer, heart disease, diabetes and scores of other major chronic diseases. It often seems as if we take two steps back for every step forward. In place of the five-dollar home remedy or the sip of brandy that often did the trick for our grandparents, we now have thousand-dollar pills and hospital bills that bankrupt families. Are these modern treatments really a thousand times better, or are there other reasons that medical expenses absorb so much of our personal and national income?

The rise in the ranks of the Medical Matrix profession has been steady and impressive. In 1900, there was one doctor for every 750 Americans; today, there are two or three per thousand, depending on the region. How and why did this growth occur, even while many of the diseases that formerly occupied our physicians have been decimated or even eradicated? Medical training at the beginning of the twentieth century generally consisted of a two-year apprenticeship, after which most doctors earned roughly the same salary as a good mechanic. With the salary of a physician so low given the demands of the profession, it was hard to recruit and retain doctors.

For the Medical Matrix industry to grow and prosper, it was essential to present the profession as a lucrative one. The man who took on this job was Dr. George H. Simmons, the homeopath editor of the *American Medical Association Journal* in 1900, who proclaimed, "The growth of the profession must be stemmed if the individual members are to find the practice of medicine a lucrative profession."

Once he decided on his goal of cutting the number of doctors in order to elevate salaries, Dr. Simmons had the great good fortune of attracting sympathy to his cause from the world's richest man, John D. Rockefeller Sr., the semiretired and notorious billionaire head of Standard Oil, who had deputized Baptist clergyman Frederick T. Gates, his most important business advisor, as his "agent for philanthropic endeavors" and was looking to get involved in the medical field. It has been suggested that John D. Rockefeller Sr., i.e., the Architect, saw the medical field not as an opportunity to distribute his largesse for the benefit of American society, but rather as a chance to increase his prestige, his wealth and his power by creating a monopoly over the health care system that had the potential to bring in more revenue than the oil business.

While this never quite came to pass during his lifetime, it must be acknowledged that the impact of Rockefeller's investments in medical research, medical education and the American hospital system represents one of his enduring legacies.

Rockefeller, like most men of his time, believed in home remedies and homeopathic medicine. He was the son of a con artist and snake oil salesman who traveled around the small-town circuit selling miracle cures. Bill Rockefeller famously bragged, "I cheat my sons every chance I get. I want to make them sharp." Ron Chernow, John D. Rockefeller's biographer, suggested that the key to understanding Rockefeller's life was to see everything he did as a reaction against his father.

By the end of his life, John D. Rockefeller had devoted more than half a billion dollars to charity. Biographer Chernow flatly calls him "the greatest philanthropist in history." The fact that much of that investment went to the causes of medical research and education rather than to the Baptist Church was in large part due to the acumen of Frederick Gates, who pushed Rockefeller in a direction that could not have been foreseen.

Rockefeller considered Frederick Gates the greatest businessman he knew, and valued him over other magnates such as Andrew Carnegie and even Henry Ford, whose promotion of the internal combustion engine arguably was the greatest single factor in making Rockefeller the richest man on earth. After being appointed head of philanthropy, Gates went right to work creating a strategy that would lay the cornerstone for the Rockefeller medical monopoly.

Gates presented Rockefeller with a plan to dominate the entire medical education system within the United States. This plan took concrete form with the creation of the Rockefeller Institute of Medical Research, still one of the world's leading medical research establishments.

The next step occurred in 1907, when the AMA requested that the Carnegie Foundation conduct a survey of all the medical schools in the country. The Carnegie Foundation appointed education reformer Abraham Flexner, who had published a critical report on the state of college education in 1908, and who is perhaps best known today as the founder of Princeton's Institute of Advanced Research, academic home to Albert Einstein in his later years, to head the study of the medical schools for the AMA. The resulting *Flexner Report* was published in 1910. Simon Flexner, Abraham's brother, who had studied pathology and then served as a professor of medicine at Johns Hopkins University, was by that time the head of the Rockefeller Institute of Medical Research. He worked closely with his brother on conducting this research on medical education.

It seems that the person who had the greatest impact on the *Flexner Report* may have been the longtime president of the

Johns Hopkins University, Daniel Coit Gilman (1831–1908), a leading member of the Rockefeller General Education Board who had recently died. Gilman had led the Carnegie Institute, a center of science education in Washington, DC, as its first president following his retirement from Johns Hopkins. Gilman believed in the German model of advanced education, and his inauguration as JHU president is often said to mark the beginning of graduate school training in the United States.

Gilman, a Yale graduate, had been an active member of the Skull and Bones Society, an elite group whose ranks have included many distinguished Americans, including both President Bushes. Gilman later cofounded the Russell Sage Foundation in order to finance the activities of Skull and Bones.

These activities, which are secret, have been construed by some to include plots to dominate the world by promoting members of the Yale elite. During the first George Bush administration, Bush's use of the catchphrase "New World Order" in reference to the opportunities presented by a post-Cold War world, was taken by some on the fundamentalist Christian right, notably former Republican candidate Pat Robertson, as a signal that Bush was a frontman for the planned establishment of an authoritarian one-world government run by the United Nations. The Persian Gulf War against Saddam Hussein's Iraq, which involved a huge coalition of countries and was financed largely by Saudi Arabia, added fuel to the fire. Now that a third Bush family member, who developed his political career as "an education reformer," has declared his interest in pursuing the presidency, with one of the chief obstacles in his path being Yale law graduate and former first lady Hillary Clinton, it is hard to avoid the impression that someone is stacking the deck in favor of the political equivalent of the Five Families!

Sinister or not, it cannot be denied that Skull and Bones alumni have been famously active in the highest reaches of American society. William Howard Taft, whose father had founded the society, was president of the United States at the time the *Flexner Report* appeared.

During Gilman's long career in education, he would act as a founder, executive officer and/or board member for many of the charitable trusts that formed the basis for what eventually became the Rockefeller Foundation. He was a trustee of the John F. Slater and Peabody Education Funds, which eventually merged with Rockefeller's Southern Education Fund to become the "General Education Fund," whose mission was to reform education across the United States. Among the pet causes of the GEF were women's education and Black education. Spelman College, one of the leading centers for the education of African American women in the United States, located in Atlanta, Georgia, is named for John D. Rockefeller's abolitionist wife, Laura Spelman Rockefeller. Rockefeller was so impressed when he first visited the college that he paid off its debt and financed the construction of its main building, now known as Rockefeller Hall. Alumni of Spelman College, which is sometimes called "the Radcliffe of the South," include novelist Alice Walker and children's advocate Marian Wright Edelman.

Gilman recruited several fellow Bonesmen to teach at the Johns Hopkins Medical School. Among these were William Henry Welch, a dominant figure in American medical education for fifty years; William Stewart Halstead, JHU's first professor of surgery, who has been called "the most important figure in the history of surgery in America"; and Harvey Williams Cushing, the pioneering neurosurgeon.

Abraham Flexner was thoroughly familiar with the German-derived Johns Hopkins educational model implemented under Gilman: JHU was Flexner's alma mater. Flexner later wrote an admiring biography of Gilman, a biography in which he carefully avoids any mention of Skull and Bones or the infamous Illuminati, with whom Gilman allegedly had deep connections.

Flexner needed no convincing on the superior merits of the German educational system. His parents had emigrated from Germany, and he had traveled and studied in Germany as a young man. The *Flexner Report* made the case that allopathic medicine and the German model of advanced clinical training offered the best hope for the future of American medicine. Conveniently, raising the standards of medical education in this way raised huge barriers to entry into the Medical Matrix profession. This was fine with Rockefeller, whose hope for a monopoly on medical education depended on weeding out competition. Flexner's conclusions were perfectly aligned with these interests: "Reckless overproduction of cheap doctors has resulted in general overcrowding. It appears, then, that the country needs fewer and better doctors; and that the way to get better is to produce fewer."

Flexner presented a solution that would make medical education so elite, expensive and drawn out that few would consider medicine as a career in the future. To achieve this purpose, Flexner set up strict requirements that consisted of four years of undergraduate college, followed by a further four years of medical school. Two-year apprenticeships would no longer suffice. The *Flexner Report* stated that Medical Matrix schools now must have expensive laboratories and equipment. As a result of the drastic changes that were implemented by the *Flexner Report*, the number of medical schools in the United States rapidly declined, from 650 to only 50 in a matter of a few years. Annual graduation numbers were reduced from 7,500 to only 2,500. This great reduction ensured that the Medical Matrix monopoly in the United States would create, by design, a very small group of elite students from affluent families.

The surprise downside for this new, small, elite group of allopathic medical doctors is that they would now be subject to intense controls, overseen by the Rockefeller Foundation in partnership with the AMA, state medical boards, and the government of the United States. Over the next few years, the AMA successfully lobbied for the creation of the United States Public Health Services, which consolidated all the public health agencies of the United States government into a single entity. This did not happen without a fight. The National League for Medical Freedom, a group lobbying for the interests of homeopaths, patent medicine sellers, and alternative healers, had successfully defeated a congressional attempt to create a large Department of Health just a year or so earlier.

The Medical Matrix's "Rockefeller Foundation" had started working on joint projects with the US Public Health Services since before the time the agency was officially chartered. This cooperation in the management of typhus, ringworm and other diseases was one of the earliest examples in the series of "public-private partnerships" that has come to dominate the landscape not only in the health care field, but even more prominently in defense contracting and procurement.

Rockefeller's good friend, the legendary financier J.P. Morgan, had single-handedly engineered the bailout of the United States government in the wake of the Panic of 1907. Within just a few years, John D. Rockefeller, who had contributed millions of dollars to Morgan's heroic effort, was able to leverage the full faith and credit of the United States on behalf of his pet projects on medical education and research.

Today, everyone knows that if you want to influence the government, you do it through a think tank; if you want to get a government grant, you apply through a foundation. In no field other than national defense are the dollars and the stakes higher than the fields of health care and education.

By co-opting the government for his purposes in the way I have described, John D. Rockefeller established a Medical Matrix system that has come to characterize the United States government more than anything that is written in the Constitution. The bottom line is that the richest man in the world figured out how to use your money to achieve his purposes, and that his family and the successors of his cronies are still making hay by his brilliant methods nearly eighty years after his death.

The United States of America today is the land of the 1 percent, a place where the rich easily evade taxes by establishing family foundations and other organizations that serve their interests. This battle has been largely waged and won on behalf of the plutocrats by having their frontmen (and women) advocate for and against health care reform. By making it all about improving medical education, expanding access to community health care, and funneling research dollars into supposedly life-saving drugs, the folks at the top of the pyramid have accumulated obscene amounts of wealth. The Medical Matrix exists because of Rockefeller's desire to profit from the pain and suffering of the American people. In 2024, it continues to exist because everyone since 1913 has been plugged in since birth. The public's continued blind faith allows for the simulation to grow and devour more money, power and control over the health, life and vitality of each generation of today and moving forward. Fear not, there is a way out!

CHAPTER 3

1969: EVIDENCE OF A SECRET MEDICAL SEMINAR TASKED TO TRANSFORM AMERICA

"The Matrix is everywhere. It's all around us. Even now, in this very room. You can see it when you look out your window, or when you turn on your television. You can feel it when you go to work, when you go to church, when you pay your taxes. It is the world that has been pulled over your eyes to blind you from the truth. You are a slave, Neo. Like everyone else you were born into bondage, born into a prison that you cannot smell or taste or touch. A prison for your mind."

– Morpheus speaking to Neo from *The Matrix* movie

1969: Dr. Lawrence Dunegan, MD, Recalling the Talk Dr. Richard Day, MD, Gave

Dr. Richard Day, MD, taught at Mount Sinai from 1968 until he retired in 1971. Earlier in his career, he was the national medical director of Planned Parenthood (1965–1968), professor and chairman of the Department of Pediatrics at the

University of Pittsburgh (1956–1965), professor and chairman of the Department of Pediatrics in the Downstate Medical School in Brooklyn (1953–1956), and associate professor at the College of Physicians and Surgeons, Columbia University (1935–1953).

Dr. Lawrence Dunegan, MD, was invited to attend a lecture given by Dr. Richard Day, MD, on March 20, 1969, to eighty to ninety medical doctors. Dr. Richard Day was an insider admitting that indeed there was an organized power group of men, who wielded enough influence to determine major events involving countries around the world, and he expounded on changes that were planned for the remainder of the twentieth century.

The following transcript is part one from the US Coalition for Life. It is a transcript of the first of three tapes on the "New Order of Barbarians," referred to on the tapes simply as the "New World System." Tapes one and two, made in 1988, are the reminiscences of Dr. Lawrence Dunegan, MD, of a speech given March 20, 1969, by Dr. Richard Day.

It's interesting to note that Dr. Dunegan "spilled the beans" in 1988. According to the bio information, Dr. Day died shortly thereafter, in 1989. It could be a coincidence since Dr. Day was elderly when he died, and then again …

Most of you reading this are very well aware, already, of many of the details involved in the diabolical plan to bring about a "New World Order" facilitated by the Medical Matrix. I believe these tapes could change many lives and awaken many more people to the reality of what lies ahead if we don't stop the process. There are many more millions of us than there are of the planners. The useful idiots—their words, not ours—who are helping the process along know not what they do. If they did know, they would stop, because they would know that they, too, will be either terminated or become part of a Matrix's "global slave camp."

Dr. Dunegan reveals not just *WHAT* is intended for America and all people in the world, but *HOW* the hidden hand of power intends to carry out their plan. He covers topics such as:

- Is there a power, a force or a group of men organizing and redirecting change?
- "Everything is in place and nobody can stop us now ..."
- People will have to get used to change—everything will change, constantly.
- The REAL and the "STATED" goals.
- Population control.
- Permission to have babies.
- Redirecting the purpose of sex—sex without reproduction and reproduction without sex.
- Sex education as a tool of World Government.
- Encouraging homosexuality, sex, anything goes.
- Euthanasia and the "demise pill."
- Limiting access to affordable medical care makes eliminating the elderly easier.
- Planning the control over medicine.
- Elimination of private doctors.
- New difficult to diagnose and untreatable diseases.

- Suppressing cancer cures as a means of population control.
- Inducing heart attacks as a form of assassination.
- Education as a tool for accelerating the onset of puberty and pushing evolution and *MUCH, MUCH MORE.*

IS THERE A POWER, A FORCE OR A GROUP OF MEN ORGANIZING AND REDIRECTING CHANGE?

There has been much written, and much said, by some people who have looked at all the changes that have occurred in American society in the past twenty years or so, and who have looked retrospectively to earlier history of the United States, and indeed, of the world, and come to the conclusion that there is a conspiracy of sorts which influences, indeed controls, major historical events, not only in the United States but around the world. This conspiratorial interpretation of history is based on people making observations from the outside, gathering evidence and coming to the conclusion that from the outside they see a conspiracy. Their evidence and conclusions are based on evidence gathered in retrospect. Period.

I want to now describe what I heard from a speaker in 1969, which in several weeks will be twenty years ago. The speaker did not speak in terms of retrospect, but rather predicting changes that would be brought about in the future. The speaker was not looking from the outside in, thinking that he saw conspiracy, rather, he was on the inside, admitting that, indeed, there was an organized power, force, group of men, who wielded enough influence to determine major events involving countries around the world. And he predicted, or rather expounded on, changes that were planned for the remainder of this century.

As you listen, if you can recall the situation, at least in the United States in 1969 and the few years thereafter, and then recall the kinds of changes which have occurred between then and now, almost twenty years later, I believe you will be impressed with the degree to which the things that were planned to be brought about have already been accomplished. Some of the things that were discussed were not intended to be accomplished yet by 1988 [Ed. Note: the year Dr. Dunegan made this tape,] but it is intended to be accomplished before the end of this century. There is a timetable, and it was during this session that some of the elements of the timetable were brought out.

Anyone who recalls early in the days of the Kennedy presidency, the Kennedy campaign, when he spoke of "progress in the decade of the '60s"; that was kind of a cliché in those days—"the decade of the '60s."

Well, by 1969 our speaker was talking about the decade of the '70s, the decade of the '80s, and the decade of the '90s. So I think that the terminology that we are looking at, looking at things and expressing things, probably all comes from the same source. Prior to that time I don't remember anybody saying "the decade of the '40s and the decade of the '50s."

So I think this overall plan and timetable had taken important shape with more predictability to those who control it, sometime in the late '50s. That's speculation on my part.

In any event, the speaker said that his purpose was to tell us about changes which would be brought about in the next thirty years or so, so that an entirely new worldwide system would be in operation before the turn of the century. As he put it, "We plan to enter the twenty-first century with a running start. Everything is in place and nobody can stop us now."

As we listened to what he was about to present he said, "Some of you will think I'm talking about communism. Well, what I'm talking about is much bigger than communism!" At that time he indicated that there is much more cooperation between East and West than most people realize. In his introductory remarks he commented that he was free to speak at this time because now, and I'm quoting here, "Everything is in place and nobody can stop us now." That's the end of that quotation. He went on to say that most people don't understand how governments operate and even people in high positions in governments, including our own, don't really understand how and where decisions are made.

He went on to say that people who really influence decisions are names that, for the most part, would be familiar to most of us, but he would not use individuals' names or names of any specific organization. But, that if he did, most of the people would be names that were recognized by most of his audience. He went on to say that they were not primarily people in public office, but people of prominence who were primarily known in their private occupations or private positions.

The speaker was a doctor of medicine, a former professor at a large Eastern university, and he was addressing a group of doctors of medicine, about eighty in number. His name would not be widely recognized by anybody likely to hear this, and so there is no point in giving his name. The only purpose in recording this is that it may give a perspective to those who hear it regarding the changes which have already been accomplished in the past twenty years or so, and a bit of a preview to what at least some people are planning for the remainder of this century so that we—or they—would enter the twenty-first century with a flying start. Some of us may not enter that century.

His purpose in telling our group about these changes that were to be brought about was to make it easier for us to adapt to these changes. Indeed, as he quite accurately said, they would be, and he hopes that we, as sort of his friends, would make the adaptation more easily if we knew somewhat beforehand what to expect.

PEOPLE WILL HAVE TO GET USED TO CHANGE

Somewhere in the introductory remarks he insisted that nobody have a tape recorder and that nobody take notes, which for a professor was a very remarkable kind of thing to expect from an audience. Something in his remarks suggested that there could be negative repercussions against him if it became widely known what he was about to say to our group, that he spilled the beans, so to speak. When I heard that, first I thought maybe that was sort of an ego trip, somebody enhancing his own importance. But as the revelations unfolded, I began to understand why he might have had some concern about not having widely known what was said, although this was a fairly public forum where he was speaking, [where the] remarks were delivered. But, nonetheless, he asked that no notes be taken, no tape recording be used suggesting there might be some personal danger to himself if these revelations were widely publicized.

Again, as the remarks began to unfold, and I saw the rather outrageous things that were said at that time, they certainly seemed outrageous, I made it a point to try to remember as much of what he said as I could, and during the subsequent weeks and months and years, to connect my recollections to simple events around me, both to aid my memory for the future in case I wanted to do what I'm doing now record this. And also, to try to maintain a perspective on what would be developing, if indeed, it followed the predicted pattern, which it has!

At this point, so that I don't forget to include it later, I'll just include some statements that were made from time to time throughout the presentation … just having a general bearing on the whole presentation. One of the statements had to do with change. The statement was, "People will have to get used to the idea of change, so used to change, that they'll be expecting change. Nothing will be permanent." This often came out in the context of a society of where people seemed to have no roots or moorings, but would be passively willing to accept change simply because it was all they had ever known. This was sort in contrast to generations of people up until this time where certain things you expected to be, and remain in place as reference points for your life. So change was to be brought about, change was to be anticipated and expected, and accepted, no questions asked.

Another comment that was made from time to time during the presentation was, "People are too trusting. People don't ask the right questions." Sometimes, being too trusting was equated with being too dumb. But sometimes when he would say that, "People don't ask the right questions," it was almost with a sense of regret, as if he were uneasy with what he was part of, and wished that people would challenge it and maybe not be so trusting.

THE REAL AND THE "STATED" GOALS

Another comment that was repeated from time to time, this particularly in relation to changing laws and customs and specific changes he said, "Everything has two purposes. One is the ostensible purpose which will make it acceptable to people; and second, is the real purpose which would further the goals of establishing the new system and having it." Frequently he would say, "There is just no other way. There's just no other way!"

This seemed to come as a sort of an apology, particularly when at the conclusion of describing some particularly offensive changes; for example, the promotion of drug addiction, which we'll get into shortly.

POPULATION CONTROL

He was very active with population control groups, the population control movement, and population control was really the entry point into specifics following the introduction. He said the population is growing too fast. The number of people living at any one time on the planet must be limited or we will run out of space to live. We will outgrow our food supply and we will over-pollute the world with our waste.

PERMISSION TO HAVE BABIES

People won't be allowed to have babies just because they want to or because they are careless. Most families would be limited to two. Some people would be allowed only one, and the outstanding person or persons might be selected and allowed to have three. But most people would [be] allowed to have only two babies. That's because the zero population growth [rate] is 2.1 children per completed family. So something like every tenth family might be allowed the privilege of the third baby.

To me, up to this point, the word "population control" primarily connoted limiting the number of babies to be born. But this remark, about what people would be "allowed" and then what followed, made it quite clear that when you hear "population control" that means more than just controlling births. It means control of every endeavor of the entire world population, a much broader meaning to that term than I had ever attached to it before hearing this. As you listen and reflect back on some of the things you hear, you will begin to recognize how one aspect dovetails with other aspects in terms of controlling human endeavors.

REDIRECTING THE PURPOSE OF SEX – SEX WITHOUT REPRODUCTION AND REPRODUCTION WITHOUT SEX

Well, from population control, the natural next step then was sex. He said sex must be separated from reproduction. Sex is too pleasurable, and the urges are too strong, to expect people to give it up. Chemicals in food and in the water supply to reduce the sex drive is not practical. The strategy then would be not to diminish sex activity, but to increase sex activity, but in such a way that people won't be having babies.

CONTRACEPTION UNIVERSALLY AVAILABLE TO ALL

And the first consideration then was contraception. Contraception would be very strongly encouraged, and it would be connected so closely in people's minds with sex, that they would automatically think of contraception when they were thinking or preparing for sex. And contraception would be made universally available. Contraceptives would be displayed much more prominently in drug stores, right up with the cigarettes and chewing gum. Out in the open, rather than hidden under the counter where people would have to ask for them and maybe be embarrassed. This kind of openness was a way of suggesting that contraceptives are just as much a part of life as any other items sold in the store. And, contraceptives would be advertised. And, contraceptives would be dispensed in the schools in association with sex education!

SEX EDUCATION AS A TOOL OF WORLD GOVERNMENT

The sex education was to get kids interested early, making the connection between sex and the need for contraception early in their lives, even before they became very active. At this point I was recalling some of my teachers, particularly in high school and found it totally unbelievable to think of them agreeing, much less participating in distributing contraceptives to students. But, that only reflected my lack of understanding of how these people operate. That was before the school-based clinic programs got started.

Many, many cities in the United States by this time have already set up school-based clinics which are primarily contraception, birth control, and population control clinics. The idea then is that the connection between sex and contraception introduced and reinforced in school would carry over into marriage. Indeed, if young people—when they matured—decided to get married, marriage itself would be diminished in importance. He indicated some recognition that most people probably would want to be married, but that this certainly would not be any longer considered to be necessary for sexual activity.

TAX FUNDED ABORTION AS POPULATION CONTROL

No surprise then, that the next item was abortion. And this, now back in 1969, four years before Roe vs. Wade. He said, "Abortion will no longer be a crime. Abortion will be accepted as 'normal,' and would be paid for by taxes for people who could not pay for their own abortions. Contraceptives would be made available by tax money so that nobody would have to do without contraceptives. If school sex programs would lead to more pregnancies in children, that was really seen as no problem. Parents who think they are opposed to abortion on moral or religious grounds will change their minds when it is their own child who is pregnant. So this will help overcome opposition to abortion. Before long, only a few die-hards will still refuse to see abortion as acceptable, and they won't matter anymore."

ENCOURAGING HOMOSEXUALITY. SEX, ANYTHING GOES

Homosexuality also was to be encouraged. "People will be given permission to be homosexual." That's the way it was stated. They won't have to hide it. And elderly people will be encouraged to continue to have active sex lives into the very old ages, just as long as they can. Everyone will be given permission to have sex, to enjoy however they want. Anything goes. This is the way it was put. And, I remember thinking, "How arrogant for this individual, or whoever he represents, to feel that they can give or withhold permission for people to do things!" But that was the terminology that was used.

In this regard, clothing was mentioned. Clothing styles would be made more stimulating and provocative. Recall back in 1969 was the time of the mini skirt, when those miniskirts were very, very high and revealing. He said, "It is not just the amount of skin that is exposed that makes clothing sexually seductive, but other, more subtle things are often suggestive," things like movement, and the cut of clothing, and the kind of fabric, the positioning of accessories on the clothing. "If a woman has an attractive body, why should she not show it?" was one of the statements.

There was no detail on what was meant by "provocative clothing," but since that time if you watched the change in clothing styles, blue jeans are cut in a way that they're more tight-fitting in the crotch. They form wrinkles. Wrinkles are essentially arrows. Lines which direct one's vision to certain anatomic areas. And, this was around the time of the "burn your bra" activity. He indicated that a lot of women should not go without a bra. They need a bra to be attractive, so instead of banning bras and burning them, bras would come back. But they would be thinner and softer allowing more natural movement. It was not specifically stated, but certainly a very thin bra is much more revealing of the nipple and what else is underneath, than the heavier bras that were in style up to that time.

Earlier he said, "Sex and reproduction would be separated." You would have sex without reproduction and then technology was reproduction without sex. This would be done in the laboratory. He indicated that already, much, much research was underway about making babies in the laboratory. There was some elaboration on that, but I don't remember the details, how much of that technology has come to my attention since that time. I don't remember in a way that I can distinguish what was said from what I subsequently have learned as general medical information.

FAMILIES TO DIMINISH IN IMPORTANCE

Families would be limited in size. We already alluded to not being allowed more than two children. Divorce would be made easier and more prevalent. Most people who marry will marry more than once. More people will not marry. Unmarried people would stay in hotels and even live together. That would be very common—nobody would even ask questions about it. It would be widely accepted as no different from married people being together.

More women will work outside the home. More men will be transferred to other cities, and in their jobs, more men will travel. Therefore, it would be harder for families to stay together. This would tend to make the marriage relationship less stable and, therefore, tend to make people less willing to have babies. And, the extended families would be smaller, and more remote. Travel would be easier, less expensive, for a while, so that people who did have to travel would feel they could get back to their families, not that they were abruptly being made remote from their families.

But one of the net effects of easier divorce laws combined with the promotion of travel, and transferring families from one city to another, was to create instability in the families. If both husband and wife are working and one partner gets transferred the other one may not be easily transferred. So one either keeps his or her job and stays behind while the other leaves, or else gives up the job and risks not finding employment in the new location. Rather a diabolical approach to this whole thing.

EUTHANASIA AND THE "DEMISE PILL"

Everybody has a right to live only so long. The old are no longer useful. They become a burden. You should be ready to accept death. Most people are. An arbitrary age limit could be established. After all, you have a right to only so many steak dinners, so many orgasms, and so many good pleasures in life. And after you have had enough of them and you're no longer productive, working, and contributing, then you should be ready to step aside for the next generation.

Some things that would help people realize that they had lived long enough, he mentioned several of these … I don't remember them all … here are a few: Use of very pale printing ink on forms that people … are necessary … to fill out, so that older people wouldn't be able to read the pale ink as easily and would need to go to younger people for help. Automobile traffic patterns—there would be more high-speed traffic lanes, traffic patterns that older people with their slower reflexes would have trouble dealing with and thus, lose some of their independence.

LIMITING ACCESS TO AFFORDABLE MEDICAL CARE, MAKES ELIMINATING THE ELDERLY EASIER

A big item that was elaborated at some length was the cost of medical care would be burdensome and high. Medical care would be connected very closely with one's work, but also would be made very, very high in cost so that it would simply be unavailable to people beyond a certain time. And unless they had a remarkably rich, supporting family, they would just have to do without care.

And the idea was that if everybody says, "Enough! What a burden it is on the young to try to maintain the old people," then the young would become agreeable to helping Mom and Dad along the way, provided this was done humanely and with dignity. And then the real example was—there could be like a nice, farewell party, a real celebration. Mom and Dad had done a good job. And then after the party's over they take the "demise pill."

PLANNING THE CONTROL OVER MEDICINE

The next topic is Medicine. There would be profound changes in the practice of medicine. Overall, medicine would be much more tightly controlled. The observation was made, "Congress is not going to go along with national health insurance. That (in 1969)," he said, "is now abundantly evident. But it's not necessary. We have other ways to control health care."

These would come about more gradually, but all health care delivery would come under tight control. Medical care would be closely connected to work. If you don't work or can't work, you won't have access to medical care. The days of hospitals giving away free care would gradually wind down, to where it was virtually nonexistent. Costs would be forced up so that people won't be able to afford to go without insurance. People pay, you pay for it, you're entitled to it. It was only subsequently that I began to realize the extent to which you would not be paying for it. Your medical care would be paid for by others. And therefore you would gratefully accept, on bended knee, what was offered to you as a privilege. Your role being responsible for your own care would be diminished.

As an aside here, this is not something that was developed at this time. I didn't understand at the time the way this works, everybody's made dependent on insurance. And if you don't have insurance then you pay directly; the cost of your care is enormous. The insurance company, however, paying for your care, does not pay that same amount. If you are charged, say, $600 on your part, they pay $300 or $400. And that differential in billing has the desired effect: It enables the insurance company to pay for that which you could never pay for. They get a discount that's unavailable to you. When you see your bill you're grateful that the insurance company could do that. And in this way you are dependent, and virtually required to have insurance. The whole billing is fraudulent.

Anyhow, continuing on now, access to hospitals would be tightly controlled. Identification would be needed to get into the building. The security in and around hospitals would be established and gradually increased so that nobody without identification could get in or move around inside the building. Theft of hospital equipment, things like typewriters and microscopes and so forth would be "allowed" and exaggerated; reports of it would be exaggerated so that this would be the excuse needed to establish the need for strict security, until people got used to it. And anybody moving about in a hospital would be required to wear an identification badge with a photograph and telling why he was there, employee or lab technician or visitor or whatever.

This is to be brought in gradually, getting everybody used to the idea of identifying themselves, until it was just accepted. This need for ID to move about would start in small ways: hospitals, some businesses, but gradually expand to include everybody in all places! It was observed that hospitals can be used to confine people for the treatment of criminals.

This did not mean, necessarily, medical treatment. At that time, I did not know the word "Psycho-Prison" as in the Soviet Union, but without trying to recall all the details, basically, he was describing the use of hospitals both for treating the sick and for confinement of criminals for reasons other than the medical well-being of the criminal. The definition of criminal was not given.

ELIMINATION OF PRIVATE DOCTORS

The image of the doctor would change. No longer would he be seen as an individual professional in service to individual patients. But the doctor would be gradually recognized as a highly skilled technician and his job would change. The job is to include things like executions by lethal injection. The image of the doctor being a powerful, independent person would have to be changed. And he went on to say, "Doctors are making entirely too much money. They should advertise like any other product."

Lawyers would be advertising too. Keep in mind, this was an audience of doctors being addressed by a doctor. And it was interesting that he would make some rather insulting statements to his audience without fear of antagonizing us. The solo practitioner would become a thing of the past. A few die-hards might try to hold out, but most doctors would be employed by an institution of one kind or another. Group practice would be encouraged, corporations would be encouraged, and then once the corporate image of medical care as this gradually became more and more acceptable, doctors would more and more become employees rather than independent contractors. And along with that, of course, unstated but necessary, is the employee serves his employer, not his patient.

So we've already seen quite a lot of that in the last twenty years. And apparently more on the horizon. The term HMO was not used at that time, but as you look at HMOs you see this is the way that medical care is being taken over since the National Health Insurance approach did not get through the

Congress. A few die-hard doctors may try to make a go of it, remaining in solo practice, remaining independent, which, parenthetically, is me. But they would suffer a great loss of income. They'd be able to scrape by, maybe, but never really live comfortably as would those who were willing to become employees of the system. Ultimately, there would be no room at all for the solo practitioner, after the system is entrenched.

NEW DIFFICULT TO DIAGNOSE AND UNTREATABLE DISEASES

Next heading to talk about is health and disease. He said there would be new diseases to appear which had not ever been seen before. Would be very difficult to diagnose and be untreatable at least for a long time. No elaboration was made on this, but I remember, not long after hearing this presentation, when I had a puzzling diagnosis to make, I would be wondering, "Is this what he was talking about? Is this a case of what he was talking about?" Some years later, as AIDS ultimately developed, I think AIDS was at least one example of what he was talking about. I now think that AIDS probably was a manufactured disease.

SUPPRESSING CANCER CURES AS A MEANS OF POPULATION CONTROL

He said, "We can cure almost every cancer right now. Information is on file in the Rockefeller Institute, if it's ever decided that it should be released. But consider—if people stop dying of cancer, how rapidly we would become overpopulated. You may as well die of cancer as something else."

Efforts at cancer treatment would be geared more toward comfort than toward cure. There was some statement that ultimately the cancer cures which were being hidden in the Rockefeller Institute would come to light because independent researchers might bring them out, despite these efforts to suppress them. But at least for the time being, letting people die of cancer was a good thing to do because it would slow down the problem of overpopulation.

INDUCING HEART ATTACKS AS A FORM OF ASSASSINATION

Another very interesting thing was heart attacks. He said, "There is now a way to simulate a real heart attack. It can be used as a means of assassinates."

Only a very skilled pathologist who knew exactly what to look for at an autopsy, could distinguish this from the real thing. I thought that was a very surprising and shocking thing to hear from this particular man at that particular time. This, and the business of the cancer cure, really still stand out sharply in my memory, because they were so shocking and, at that time, seemed to me out of character.

He then went on to talk about nutrition and exercise, sort of in the same framework. People would not have to eat right and exercise right to live as long as before. Most won't. Thus, in the connection of nutrition, there was no specific statement that I can recall as to particular nutrients that would be either inadequate or in excess. In retrospect, I tend to think he meant high-salt diets and high-fat diets would predispose toward high blood pressure and premature arteriosclerotic heart disease. And that if people who were too dumb or too lazy to exercise as they should then have their dietary and their circulating fats go up and predispose to disease.

And he said something about diet information about proper diet would be widely available, but most people, particularly stupid people, who had no right to continue living anyway they would ignore the advice and just go on and eat what was convenient and tasted good. There were some other unpleasant things said about food. I just can't recall what they were. But I do remember having reflections about wanting to plant a garden in the backyard to get around whatever these contaminated foods would be. I regret I don't remember the details, the rest of this, about nutrition and hazardous nutrition.

With regard to exercise. He went on to say that more people would be exercising more, especially running, because everybody can run. You don't need any special equipment or place. You can run wherever you are. As he put it, "People will be running all over the place." And in this vein, he pointed out how supply produces demand. And this was in reference to athletic clothing and equipment. As this would be made more widely available and glamorized, particularly as regards running shoes, this would stimulate people to develop an interest in running and as part of a whole sort of public propaganda campaign, people would be encouraged then to buy the attractive sports equipment and to get into exercise.

Again, well in connection with nutrition he also mentioned that public eating places would rapidly increase. That this had a connection with the family too. As more and more people eat out, eating at home would become less important. People would be less dependent on their kitchens at home. And then this also connected to convenience foods being made widely available, things like you could pop into the microwave. Whole meals would be available pre-fixed. And of course, we've now seen this and some pretty good ones.

But this whole different approach to eating out and to previously prepared meals being eaten in the home was predicted at that time to be brought about convenience foods. The convenience foods would be part of the hazards. Anybody who was lazy enough to want the convenience foods rather than fixing his own also had better be energetic enough to exercise. Because if he was too lazy to exercise and too lazy to fix his own food, then he didn't deserve to live very long.

This was all presented as sort of a moral judgment about people and what they should do with their energies. People who are smart, who learn about nutrition, and who are disciplined enough to eat right and exercise right are better people and the kind you want to live longer.

EDUCATION AS A TOOL FOR ACCELERATING THE ONSET OF PUBERTY AND EVOLUTION

Somewhere along there was also something about accelerating the onset of puberty. And this was said in connection with health, and later in connection with education, and connecting to accelerating the process of evolutionary change. There was a statement that "we think that we can push evolution faster and in the direction we want it to go." I remember this only as a general statement. I don't recall if any details were given beyond that.

BLENDING ALL RELIGIONS – THE OLD RELIGIONS WILL HAVE TO GO

Another area of discussion was RELIGION. This is an avowed atheist speaking. And he said, "Religion is not necessarily bad. A lot of people seem to need religion, with its mysteries and rituals—so they will have religion." But the major religions of today have to be changed because they are not compatible with the changes to come. The old religions will have to go. Especially Christianity. Once the Roman Catholic Church is brought down, the rest of Christianity will follow easily. Then a new religion can be accepted for use all over the world. It will incorporate something from all of the old ones to make it more easy for people to accept it, and feel at home in it. Most people won't be too concerned with religion. They will realize that they don't need it.

CHANGING THE BIBLE THROUGH REVISIONS OF KEY WORDS

In order to do this, the Bible will be changed. It will be rewritten to fit the new religion. Gradually, keywords will be replaced with new words having various shades of meaning. Then, the meaning attached to the new word can be close to the old word. And as time goes on, other shades of meaning of that word can be emphasized, and then gradually that word is replaced with another word.

I don't know if I'm making that clear. But the idea is that everything in Scripture need not be rewritten, just key words replaced by other words. And the variability in meaning attached to any word can be used as a tool to change the entire meaning of Scripture, and therefore make it acceptable to this new religion. Most people won't know the difference, and this was another one of the times where he said, "The few who do notice the difference won't be enough to matter."

THE CHURCHES WILL HELP

Then followed one of the most surprising statements of the whole presentation: He said, "Some of you probably think the churches won't stand for this," and he went on to say, "The churches will help us!" There was no elaboration on this; it was unclear just what he had in mind when he said, "The churches will help us!" In retrospect, I think some of us now can understand what he might have meant at that time. I recall then only thinking, "No they won't!" and remembering our Lord's words where he said to Peter, "Thou art Peter and upon this rock I will build my Church, and gates of Hell will not prevail against it." So yes, some people in the churches might help. And in the subsequent twenty years we've seen how some people in churches have helped. We also know that our Lord's words will stand, and the gates of Hell will NOT prevail.

RESTRUCTURING EDUCATION AS A TOOL OF INDOCTRINATION

Another area of discussion was education. And one of the things in connection with education that I remember connecting with what he said about religion, was in addition to changing the Bible he said that the classics in Literature would be changed. I seem to recall Mark Twain's writings were given as one example. But he said, the casual reader reading a revised version of a classic would never even suspect that there was any change. And, somebody would have to go through word by word to even recognize that any change was made in these classics; the changes would be so subtle. But the changes would be such as to promote the acceptability of the new system.

MORE TIME IN SCHOOLS, BUT THEY "WOULDN'T LEARN ANYTHING."

As regards education, he indicated that kids would spend more time in schools, but in many schools they wouldn't learn anything. They'll learn some things, but not as much as before. Better schools in better areas with better people—their kids will learn more. In the better schools, learning would be accelerated. And this is another time where he said, "We think we can push evolution."

By pushing kids to learn more, he seemed to be suggesting that their brains would evolve, that their offspring would evolve, sort of pushing evolution where kids would learn and be more intelligent at a younger age. As if this pushing would alter their physiology.

Overall, schooling would be prolonged. This meant prolonged through the school year. I'm not sure what he said about a long school day, I do remember he said that school was planned to go all summer, that the summer school vacation would become a thing of the past. Not only for schools, but for other reasons. People would begin to think of vacation times year-round, not just in the summer.

For most people, it would take longer to complete their education. To get what originally had been in a bachelor's program would now require advanced degrees and more schooling. So that a lot of school time would be just wasted time. Good schools would become more competitive. I inferred when he said that, that he was including all schools, elementary up through college, but I don't recall whether he said that. Students would have to decide at a younger age what they would want to study and get onto their track early, if they would qualify. It would be harder to change to another field of study once you get started.

Studies would be concentrated in much greater depth, but narrowed. You wouldn't have access to material in other fields, outside your own area of study, without approval. This seems to be more where he talked about limited access to other fields. I seem to recall that as being more at the college level, high school and college level, perhaps. People would be very specialized in their own area of expertise. But they won't be able to get a broad education and won't be able to understand what is going on overall.

CONTROLLING WHO HAS ACCESS TO INFORMATION

He was already talking about computers in education, and at that time he said anybody who wanted computer access, or access to books that were not directly related to their field of study would have to have a very good reason for doing so. Otherwise, access would be denied.

SCHOOLS AS THE HUB OF THE COMMUNITY

Another angle was that the schools would become more important in people's overall life. Kids in addition to their academics, would have to get into school activities unless they wanted to feel completely out of it. But spontaneous activities among kids, the thing that came to my mind when I heard this was sandlot football and sandlot baseball teams that we worked up as kids growing up. I said the kids wanting any activities outside of school would be almost forced to get them through the school. There would be few opportunities outside.

Now the pressures of the accelerated academic program, the accelerated demands, where kids would feel they had to be part of something one or another athletic club or some school activity these pressures he recognized would cause some students to burn out. He said, "The smartest ones will learn how to cope with pressures and to survive. There will be some help available to students in handling stress, but the unfit won't be able to make it. They will then move on to other things."

In this connection, and later on in the connection with drug abuse and alcohol abuse, he indicated that psychiatric services to help would be increased dramatically. In all the pushing for achievement, it was recognized that many people would need help, and the people worth keeping around would be able to accept and benefit from that help, and still be super-achievers.

Those who could not would fall by the wayside and therefore were sort of dispensable, "expendable," I guess is the word I want. Education would be lifelong. Adults would be going to school. There'll always be new information that adults must have to keep up. When you can't keep up anymore, you're too old. This was another way of letting older people know that the time had come for them to move on and take the demise pill. If you get too tired to keep up with your education, or you get too old to learn new information, then this is a signal you begin to prepare to get ready to step aside.

SOME BOOKS WOULD JUST DISAPPEAR FROM THE LIBRARIES

In addition to revising the classics, which I alluded to a while ago with revising the Bible, he said, "Some books would just disappear from the libraries." This was in the vein that some books contain information or contain ideas that should not be kept around. And therefore, those books would disappear. I don't remember exactly if he said how this was to be accomplished. But I seem to recall carrying away this idea that this would include thefts. That certain people would be designated to go to certain libraries and pick up certain books and just get rid of them. Not necessarily as a matter of policy, just simply steal it. Further down the line, not everybody will be allowed to own books. And some books NOBODY will be allowed to own.

CHANGING LAWS

Another area of discussion was laws that would be changed. At that time a lot of States had blue laws about Sunday sales, certain Sunday activities. He said the blue laws would all be repealed. Gambling laws would be repealed or relaxed, so that gambling would be increased. He indicated then that governments would get into gambling. We've had a lot of state lotteries pop up around the country since then. And, at the time, we were already being told that would be the case. "Why should all that gambling money be kept in private hands when the State would benefit from it?" was the rationale behind it. But people should be able to gamble if they want to.

So it would become a civil activity, rather than a private, or illegal activity. Bankruptcy laws would be changed. I don't remember the details, but just that they would be changed. And I know subsequent to that time they have been. Antitrust laws would be changed, or be interpreted differently, or both. In connection with the changing antitrust laws, there was some statement that in a sense, competition would be increased. But this would be increased competition within otherwise controlled circumstances. So it's not a free competition. I recall having the impression that it was like competition but within members of a club. There would be nobody outside the club would be able to compete. Sort of like teams competing within a professional league, if you're the NFL or the American or National Baseball Leagues, you compete within the league but the league is all in agreement on what the rules of competition are not a really free competition.

ENCOURAGEMENT OF DRUG ABUSE TO CREATE A JUNGLE ATMOSPHERE

Drug use would be increased. Alcohol use would be increased. Law enforcement efforts against drugs would be increased. On first hearing that, it sounded like a contradiction. Why increase drug abuse and simultaneously increase law enforcement against drug abuse? But the idea is that, in part, the increased availability of drugs would provide a sort of law of the jungle whereby the weak and the unfit would be selected out. There was a statement made at the time: "Before the earth was overpopulated, there was a law of the jungle where only the fittest survived."

You had to be able to protect yourself against the elements and wild animals and disease. And if you were fit, you survived. But now we've become so civilized we're over-civilized and the unfit are enabled to survive, only at the expense of those who are more fit. And the abusive drugs then, would restore, in a certain sense, the law of the jungle, and selection of the fittest for survival. News about drug abuse and law enforcement efforts would tend to keep drugs in the public consciousness. And would also tend to reduce this unwarranted American complacency that the world is a safe place, and a nice place.

ALCOHOL ABUSE

The same thing would happen with alcohol. Alcohol abuse would be both promoted and demoted at the same time. The vulnerable and the weak would respond to the promotions and, therefore, use and abuse more alcohol. Drunk driving would become more of a problem, and stricter rules about driving under the influence would be established so that more and more people would lose their privilege to drive.

RESTRICTIONS ON TRAVEL

This also had connection with something we'll get to later about overall restrictions on travel. Not everybody should be free to travel the way they do now in the United States. People don't have a need to travel that way. It's a privilege! It was kind of a high-handed way it was put. Again, much more in the way of psychological services would be made available to help those who got hooked on drugs and alcohol. The idea being, that in order to promote this drug and alcohol abuse to screen out some of the unfit people who are otherwise pretty good would also be subject to getting hooked. And if they were really worth their salt they would have enough sense to seek psychological counseling and to benefit from it. So this was presented as sort of a redeeming value on the part of the planners. It was as if he were saying, "You think we're bad at promoting these evil things, but look how nice we are, we're also providing a way out!"

THE NEED FOR MORE JAILS, AND USING HOSPITALS AS JAILS

More jails would be needed. Hospitals could serve as jails. Some new hospital construction would be designed so as to make them adaptable to jail-like use.

Source/Reference: US Coalition for Life, Box 315, Export, Penn 15632

CHAPTER 4

THE SYSTEM ENGAGED: THEIR GREAT RESET AGENDA

"The Matrix is a system, Neo. That system is your enemy. But when you're inside, you look around, what do you see? Businessmen, doctors, teachers, lawyers, carpenters. The very minds of the people we are trying to save. But until we do, these people are still part of that system, and that makes them our enemy. You have to understand, most of these people are not ready to be unplugged and many of them are so injured, so hopelessly dependent on the system, that they will fight to protect it."

– Morpheus speaking to Neo from *The Matrix* movie

This is a transcript of the second of three tapes on the "New Order of Barbarians," referred to on the tapes simply as the "New World System." Tapes one and two, made in 1988, are the reminiscences of Dr. Lawrence Dunegan, MD, a pediatrician from Pittsburgh, who sat through a talk in 1969, while insider, Dr. Richard Day, MD, spoke of the planned future of America and Americans. Dr. Day was speaking to a group of pediatric physicians who were told, "No note-taking and no tape recorders."

CHANGE

Change, nothing is permanent. Streets would be rerouted, renamed. Areas you had not seen in a while would become unfamiliar. Among other things, this would contribute to older people feeling that it was time to move on, they feel they couldn't even keep up with the changes in areas that were once familiar. Buildings would be allowed to stand empty and deteriorate, and streets would be allowed to deteriorate in certain localities.

The purpose of this was to provide the jungle, the depressed atmosphere for the unfit. Somewhere in this same connection he mentioned that buildings and bridges would be made so that they would collapse after a while; there would be more accidents involving airplanes and railroads and automobiles. All of this contributed to the feeling of insecurity, that nothing was safe.

Not too long after this presentation, and I think one or two even before in the area where I live, we had some newly constructed bridge to break; another newly constructed bridge defect discovered before it broke, and I remember reading just scattered incidents around the country where shopping malls would fall in—right where they were filled with shoppers. And I remember that one of the shopping malls in our area, the first building I'd ever been in where you could feel this vibration throughout the entire building when there were a lot of people in there, and I remember wondering at that time whether this shopping mall was one of the buildings he was talking about. Talking to construction people and architects about it they would say, "Oh no, that's good when the building vibrates like that. That means it's flexible, not rigid." Well, maybe so. We'll wait and see.

Other areas there would be well maintained. Not every part of the city would be slums. There would be the created slums and other areas well maintained. Those people able to leave the slums for better areas then would learn to better appreciate the importance of human accomplishment. This meant that if they left the jungle and came to civilization, so to speak, they could be proud of their own accomplishments that they made. There was no related sympathy for those who were left behind in the jungle of drugs and deteriorating neighborhoods. Then a statement that was kind of surprising: "We think we can effectively limit crime to the slum areas, so it won't be spread heavily into better areas."

CONSOLIDATING POLICY

I should maybe point out here that these are obviously not word-for-word quotations after twenty years, but when I say that I am quoting, I am giving the general drift of what was said close to word for word, perhaps not precisely so. But anyhow, I remember wondering, "How can he be so confident that the criminal element is going to stay where he wants it to stay?" But he went on to say that increased security would be needed in the better areas.

That would mean more police, better-coordinated police efforts. He did not say so, but I wondered at that time about the moves that were afoot to consolidate all the police departments of suburbs around the major cities. I think the John Birch Society was one that was saying, "Support your local police; don't let them be consolidated." And I remember wondering if that was one of the things he had in mind about security. It was not explicitly stated. But anyhow, he went on to say there would be a whole new industry of residential security systems to develop with alarms and locks and alarms going into the police department so that people could protect their wealth and their well-being. Because some of the criminal activity would spill out of the slums into better, more affluent looking areas that looked like they would be worth burglarizing. And again it was stated like it was a redeeming quality. "See, we're generating all this more crime, but look how good we are—we're also generating the means for you to protect yourself against the crime." A sort of repeated thing throughout this presentation was the recognized evil and then the self-forgiveness thing, "Well see, we've given you a way out."

GLOBAL INTERDEPENDENCE "TO CREATE A NEW STRUCTURE, YOU FIRST HAVE TO TEAR DOWN THE OLD"

American industry came under discussion, it was the first that I'd heard the term "Global Interdependence." The stated plan was that different parts of the world would be assigned different roles of industry and commerce in a unified global system. The continued preeminence of the United States and the relative independence and self-sufficiency of the United States would have to be changed.

This was one of the several times that he said in order to create a new structure, you first have to tear down the old, and American industry was one example of that. Our system would have to be curtailed in order to give other countries a chance to build their industries, because otherwise they would not be able to compete against the United States. And this was especially true of our heavy industries that would be cut back while the same industries were being developed in other countries, notably Japan.

PATRIOTISM WOULD GO DOWN THE DRAIN

And at this point there was some discussion of steel and particularly automobiles. I remember him saying that automobiles would be imported from Japan on an equal footing with our own domestically produced automobiles, but the Japanese product would be better. Things would be made so they would break and fall apart that is, in the United States so that people would tend to prefer the imported variety and this would give a bit of a boost to foreign competitors.

One example was Japanese. In 1969, Japanese automobiles, if they were sold here at all, I don't remember, but they certainly weren't very popular. But the idea was, you could get a little bit disgusted with your Ford, GM, or Chrysler product—or whatever—because little things like window handles would fall off more, and plastic parts would break which, had they been made of metal, would hold up. Your patriotism about buying American would soon give way to practicality that if you bought Japanese, German, or imported that it would last longer and you would be better off. Patriotism would go down the drain then.

It was mentioned elsewhere, things being made to fall apart too. I don't remember specific items or if they were even stated other than automobiles, but I do recall having the impression, sort of in my imagination, of a surgeon having something fall apart in his hands in the operating room, at a critical time. Was he including this sort of thing in his discussion? But somewhere in this discussion about things being made deliberately defective and unreliable not only was to tear down patriotism but to be just a little source of irritation to people who would use such things.

LOSS OF JOBS – LOSS OF SECURITY

Again, the idea that you do not feel terribly secure, promoting the notion that the world isn't a terribly reliable place. The United States was to be kept strong in information, communications, high technology, education and agriculture. The United States was seen as continuing to be sort of the keystone of this global system. But heavy industry would be transported out. One of the comments made about heavy industry was that we had had enough environmental damage from smokestacks and industrial waste and some of the other people could put up with that for a while. This again, was supposed to be a "redeeming quality" for Americans to accept. You took away our industry but you saved our environment. So we really didn't lose on it.

POPULATION SHIFTS TO ELIMINATE "TRADITIONS"

And along this line there were talks about people losing their jobs as a result of industry and opportunities for retraining, and particularly population shifts would be brought about. This is sort of an aside. I think I'll explore the aside before I forget it. Population shifts were to be brought about so that people would be tending to move into the Sun Belt. They would be, sort of, people without roots in their new locations, and traditions are easier to change in a place where there are a lot of transplanted people, as compared to trying to changing traditions in a place where people grew up and had an extended family where they had roots. Things like new medical care systems. If you pick up from a Northeast industrial city and you transplant yourself to the South Sun Belt or Southwest, you'll be more accepting of whatever kind of, for example, controlled medical care you find there than you would accept a change in the medical care system where you had roots and the support of your family. Also in this vein it was mentioned he used the plural personal pronoun "we," we take control first of the port cities, New York, San Francisco, Seattle, the idea being that this is a piece of strategy.

The idea being that if you control the port cities with your philosophy and your way of life, the heartland in between has to yield. I can't elaborate more on that but it is interesting, if you look around the most liberal areas of the country and progressively so are the seacoast cities; the heartland, the Midwest, does seem to have maintained its conservatism. But as you take away industry and jobs and relocate people then this is a strategy to break down conservatism. When you take away industry, and people are unemployed and poor they will accept whatever change seems to offer them survival, and their morals and their commitment to things will all give way to survival. That's not my philosophy. That's the speaker's philosophy.

WORLD CITIZENS – WORLD SPORTS

Anyhow, going back to industry. Some heavy industry would remain. Just enough to maintain a sort of seedbed of industrial skills which could be expanded if the plan didn't work out as it was intended. So the country would not be devoid of assets and skills. But this was just sort of a contingency plan. It was hoped and expected that the worldwide specialization would be carried on.

But, perhaps repeating myself, one of the upsides of all of this is that with this global interdependence then national identities would tend to be de-emphasized. Each area depended on every other area for one or another element in its life. We would all become citizens of the world rather than citizens of any one country.

And along these lines then we can talk about sports. Sports in the United States was to be changed, in part as a way of de-emphasizing nationalism. Soccer, a worldwide sport, was to be emphasized and pushed in the United States and this was of interest because in this area the game of soccer was virtually unknown at that time. I had a few friends who attended an elementary school other than the one I attended where they played soccer at their school, and they were a real novelty. This was back in the '50s. So to hear this man speak of soccer in this area was kind of surprising.

Anyhow, soccer is seen as an international sport and would be promoted and the traditional sport of American baseball would be de-emphasized and possibly eliminated because it might be seen as too American. And he discussed eliminating this. One's first reaction would be well, they pay the players poorly and they don't want to play for poor pay so they give up baseball and either go into some other sport or some other activity. But, he said that's really not how it works. Actually, the way to break down baseball would be to make the salaries go very high.

The idea behind this was that as the salaries got ridiculously high there would be a certain amount of discontent and antagonism as people resented the athletes being paid so much, and the athletes would begin more and more to resent among themselves what other players were paid and would tend to abandon the sport. And these high salaries then also could break the owners and alienate the fans. And then the fans would support soccer and the baseball fields could be used as soccer fields. It wasn't said definitely this would have to happen, but if the international flavor didn't come around rapidly enough this could be done.

There was some comment along the same lines about football, although I seem to recall he said football would be harder to dismantle because it was so widely played in colleges as well as in the professional leagues and would be harder to tear down. There was something else also about the violence in football that met a psychological need that was perceived, and people have a need for this vicarious violence. So football, for that reason, might be left around to meet that vicarious need.

The same thing is true of hockey. Hockey had more of an international flavor and would be emphasized. There was some foreseeable international competition about hockey and particularly soccer. At that time hockey was international between the United States and Canada. I was kind of surprised because I thought the speaker just never impressed me as being at all a hockey fan, and I am. And it turns out, he was not. He just knew about the game and what it would do to this changing sports Program.

But in any event soccer was to be the keystone of athletics because it is already a worldwide sport in South America, in Europe, in parts of Asia and the United States should get on the bandwagon. All this would foster international competition so that we would all become citizens of the world to a greater extent than citizens of our narrow nations.

HUNTING

There was some discussion about hunting, not surprisingly. Hunting requires guns and gun control is a big element in these plans. I don't remember the details much, but the idea is that gun ownership is a privilege and not everybody should have guns. Hunting was an inadequate excuse for owning guns and everybody should be restricted in gun ownership. The few privileged people who should be allowed to hunt could maybe rent or borrow a gun from official quarters rather than own their own. After all, everybody doesn't have a need for a gun, is the way it was put.

SPORTS FOR GIRLS – TO DE-EMPHASIZE FEMININITY

Very important in sports was sports for girls. Athletics would be pushed for girls. This was intended to replace dolls. Baby dolls would still be around, a few of them, but you would not see the number and variety of dolls. Dolls would not be pushed because girls should not be thinking about babies and reproduction. Girls should be out on the athletic field just as the boys are. Girls and boys really need not to be all that different. Tea sets were to go the way of dolls, and all these things that traditionally were thought of as feminine would be de-emphasized as girls got into more masculine pursuits.

Just one other thing I recall was that the sports pages would be full of the scores of girls' teams just right along with the boys' teams. And that's recently begun to appear after twenty years in our local papers. The girls' sports scores are right along with the boys' sports scores. So all of this to change the role model of what young girls should look to be. While she's growing up she should look to be an athlete rather to look forward to being a mother.

ENTERTAINMENT: VIOLENCE, SEX AND MORE SEX DESENSITIZATION – PREPARING THE PEOPLE FOR "HUMAN CASUALTIES"

Movies would gradually be made more explicit as regards sex and language. After all, sex and rough language are real and why pretend that they are not? There would be pornographic movies in the theaters, on television. And VCRs were not around at that time, but he had indicated that these cassettes would be available, and video cassette players would be available for use in the home and pornographic movies would be available for use on these VCRs as well as in the neighborhood theater and on your television. He said something like, "You'll see people in the movies doing everything you can think of."

He went on to say that all of this is intended to bring sex out in the open. That was another comment that was made several times the term "sex out in the open." Violence would be made more graphic.

This was intended to desensitize people to violence. There might need to be a time when people would witness real violence and be a part of it. Later on it will become clear where this is headed. So there would be more realistic violence in entertainment, which would make it easier for people to adjust.

People's attitudes towards death would change and they would not be so fearful of it but more accepting of it, and not be so aghast at the sight of dead people or injured people. We don't need to have a genteel population paralyzed by what they might see. People would just learn to say, "Well, I don't want that to happen to me." This was the first statement suggesting that the plan includes numerous human casualties which the survivors would see. This particular aspect of the presentation came back in my memory very sharply a few years later when a movie about the Lone Ranger came out and I took my very young son to see it and early in the movie were some very violent scenes. One of the victims was shot in the forehead and there was sort of a splat where the bullet entered his forehead and blood and I remember regretting that I took my son, and remember feeling anger toward the doctor who spoke. Not that he made the movie, but he agreed to be part of this movement, and I was repelled by the movie and it brought back this aspect of his presentation very sharply in my memory.

MUSIC WILL GET WORSE

As regards music, he made a rather straightforward statement like, "Music will get worse." In 1969, Rock music was getting more and more unpleasant. It was interesting just his words the way he expressed it. It would "get worse," acknowledging that it was already bad. Lyrics would become more openly sexual. No new sugary romantic music would be publicized like that which had been written before that time.

All of the old music would be brought back on certain radio stations and records for older people to hear. And all the folks would have sort of their own radio stations to hear. As it got worse and worse, he seemed to indicate that one group would not hear the other group's music. Older folks would just refuse to hear the junk that was offered to young people, and the young people would accept the junk because it identified them as their generation and helped them feel distinct from the older generation.

I remember at the time thinking that would not last very long because even young kids wouldn't like the junk when they got a chance to hear the older music that was prettier they would gravitate toward it. Unfortunately, I was wrong about that, when the kids get through their teens and into their twenties some of them improve their taste in music, but unfortunately he was right. They get used to this junk and that's all they want. A lot of them can't stand really pretty music. He went on to say that the music would carry a message to the young and nobody would even know the message was there.

They would just think it was loud music. At the time, I didn't quite understand what he meant by that, but in retrospect, I think we now know what the messages are in the music for the young.

GIVE US THE YOUNG

And again, he was right. This aspect was sort of summarized with the notion that entertainment would be a tool to influence young people. It won't change the older people, they are already set in their ways, but the changes would be all aimed at the young, who are in their formative years, and the older generation would be passing. Not only could you not change them, but they are relatively unimportant, anyhow. Once they live out their lives and are gone, the younger generation being formed, are the ones that would be important for the future in the twenty-first century.

He also indicated all the old movies would be brought back again, and I remember on hearing that through my mind quickly the memories of a number of old movies. I wondered if they would be included, the ones that I thought I would like to see again. Along with bringing back old music and old movies for older people there were other privileges that would also be accorded older folks: free transportation, breaks on purchases, discounts, tax discounts, a number of privileges just because they were older. This was stated to be sort of a reward for the generation which had grown up through the depression and had survived the rigors of World War II. They had deserved it, and they were going to be rewarded with all these goodies, and the bringing back of the good old music and the good old movies were going to help ease them through their final years in comfort.

THE '80s AND '90s – THE GRIM REAPER. TRAVEL RESTRICTIONS – NATIONAL ID – THE CHIP, ETC.

Then, the presentation began to get rather grim, because once that generation passed, and that would be in the late '80s and early '90s where we are now, most of that [age] group would be gone and then, gradually, things would tighten up and the tightening up would be accelerated. The old movies and old songs would be withdrawn; the gentler entertainment would be withdrawn. Travel, instead of being easy for old folks, would become very restricted. People would need permission to travel and they would need a good reason to travel. If you didn't have a good reason for your travel you would not be allowed to travel, and everyone would need ID.

This would at first be an ID card you would carry on your person and you must show when you are asked for it. It was already planned that later on some sort of device would be developed to be implanted under the skin that would be coded specifically to identify the individual. This would eliminate the possibility of false ID and also eliminate the possibility of people saying, "Well, I lost my ID." The difficulty about these skin-implanted IDs was stated to be getting material that would stay in or under the skin without causing foreign body reaction whereby the body would reject it or cause infection, and that this would have to be material on which information could be recorded and retrieved by some sort of scanner while it was not rejected by the body.

Silicon was mentioned. Silicon at that time was thought to be well tolerated. It was used to augment breasts. Women who felt their breasts were too small would get silicone implants, and I guess that still goes on. At any rate silicon was seen at that time as the promising material to do both to be retained in the body without rejection and to be able to retain information retrievable by electronic means.

FOOD CONTROL

Food supplies would come under tight control. If population growth didn't slow down, food shortages could be created in a hurry and people would realize the dangers of overpopulation. Ultimately, whether the population slows down or not the food supply is to be brought under centralized control so that people would have enough to be well nourished but they would not have enough to support any fugitive from the new system. And growing one's own food would be outlawed. This would be done under some sort of pretext. In the beginning, I mentioned there were two purposes for everything, one the ostensible purpose and one the real purpose and the ostensible purpose here would be that growing your own vegetables was unsafe, it would spread disease or something like that.

So the acceptable idea was to protect the consumer but the real idea was to limit the food supply and growing your own food would be illegal. And if you persist in illegal activities like growing your own food, then you're a criminal.

WEATHER CONTROL

There was a mention then of weather. This was another really striking statement. He said, "We can or soon will be able to control the weather." He said, "I'm not merely referring to dropping iodide crystals into the clouds to precipitate rain that's already there, but REAL control." And weather was seen as a weapon of war, a weapon of influencing public policy. It could make rain or withhold rain in order to influence certain areas and bring them under your control. There were two sides to this that were rather striking.

He said, "On the one hand you can make drought during the growing season so that nothing will grow, and on the other hand you can make for very heavy rains during harvest season so the fields are too muddy to bring in the harvest, and indeed one might be able to do both." There was no statement how this would be done. It was stated that either it was already possible or very close to being possible.

POLITICS

He said that very few people really know how the government works. Something to the effect that elected officials are influenced in ways that they don't even realize, and they carry out plans that have been made for them, and they think that they are authors of the plans. But actually they are manipulated in ways they don't understand.

KNOW HOW PEOPLE RESPOND – MAKING THEM DO WHAT YOU WANT

Somewhere in the presentation he made two statements that I want to insert at this time. I don't remember just where they were made, but they're valid in terms of the general overall view. One statement: "People can carry in their minds and act upon two contradictory ideas at one time, provided that these two contradictory ideas are kept far enough apart."

And the other statement is, "You can know pretty well how rational people are going to respond to certain circumstances or to certain information that they encounter. So, to determine the response you want, you need only control the kind of data or information that they're presented or the kinds of circumstances that they're in, and being rational people they'll do what you want them to do. They may not fully understand what they're doing or why."

FALSIFIED SCIENTIFIC RESEARCH

Somewhere in this connection, then, was the statement admitting that some scientific research data could be and indeed HAS been falsified in order to bring about desired results. And here it was said, "People don't ask the right questions. Some people are too trusting."

Now this was an interesting statement because the speaker and the audience are all being doctors of medicine and supposedly very objectively, dispassionately scientific, and science being the be-all and end-all, well to falsify scientific research data in that setting is like blasphemy in the church … you just don't do that. Anyhow, out of all of this was to come the "New International Governing Body," probably to come through the UN and with a World Court, but not necessarily through those structures. It could be brought about in other ways.

ACCEPTANCE OF THE UN – THE END JUSTIFIES THE MEANS

Acceptance of the UN at that time was seen as not being as wide as was hoped. Efforts would continue to give the United Nations increasing importance. People would be more and more used to the idea of relinquishing some national sovereignty. Economic interdependence would foster this goal from a peaceful standpoint.

Avoidance of war would foster it from the standpoint of worrying about hostilities. It was recognized that doing it peaceably was better than doing it by war. It was stated at this point that war was "obsolete." I thought that was an interesting phrase because obsolete means something that once was seen as useful is no longer useful. But war is obsolete because of the nuclear bombs. War is no longer controllable. Formerly, wars could be controlled, but if nuclear weapons would fall into the wrong hands there could be an unintended nuclear disaster. It was not stated who the "wrong hands" are. We were free to infer that maybe this meant terrorists, but in more recent years I'm wondering whether the wrong hands might also include people that we've assumed that they've had nuclear weapons all along maybe they don't have them.

Just as it was stated that industry would be preserved in the United States a little bit, just in case the worldwide plans didn't work out; just in case some country or some other powerful person decided to bolt from the pack and go his own way one wonders whether this might also be true with nuclear weapons. When you hear that he said they might fall into the wrong hands, there was some statement that the possession of nuclear weapons had been tightly controlled, sort of implying that anybody who had nuclear weapons was intended to have them. That would necessarily have included the Soviet Union, if indeed they have them.

But I recall wondering at the time, "Are you telling us, or are you implying that this country willingly gave weapons to the Soviets?" At that time that seemed like a terribly unthinkable thing to do, much less to admit. The leaders of the Soviet Union seem to be so dependent on the West though, one wonders whether there may have been some fear that they would try to assert independence if they indeed had these weapons. So, I don't know. It's something to speculate about perhaps. Who did he mean when he said, "If these weapons fall into the wrong hands"? Maybe just terrorists.

Anyhow, the new system would be brought in, if not by peaceful cooperation everybody willingly yielding national sovereignty then by bringing the nation to the brink of nuclear war. And everybody would be so fearful as hysteria is created by the possibility of nuclear war that there would be a strong public outcry to negotiate a public peace and people would willingly give up national sovereignty in order to achieve peace, and thereby this would bring in the New International Political System.

This was stated and a very impressive thing to hear then, "If there were too many people in the right places who resisted this, there might be a need to use one or two possibly more nuclear weapons." As it was put this would be possibly needed to convince people that "We mean business."

That was followed by the statement that, "By the time one or two of those went off then everybody, even the most reluctant would yield." He said something about "this negotiated peace would be very convincing," as kind of in a framework or in a context that the whole thing was rehearsed but nobody would know it. People hearing about it would be convinced that it was a genuine negotiation between hostile enemies who finally had come to the realization that peace was better than war.

WAR IS GOOD – YOU GET TO BE CANNON FODDER, KEEP THE POPULATION DOWN, AND DIE A HERO

In this context discussing war, and war is obsolete, a statement was made that there were some good things about war one, you're going to die anyway, and people sometimes in war get a chance to display great courage and heroism and if they die they've died well and if they survive they get recognition. So that in any case, the hardships of war on soldiers are worth it because that's the reward they get out of their warring.

Another justification expressed for war was, if you think of the many millions of casualties in WWI and WWII, we'll suppose all those people had not died but had continued to live, then continued to have babies. There would be millions upon millions and we would already be overpopulated, so those two great wars served a benign purpose in delaying overpopulation. But now there are technological means for the individual and governments to control overpopulation so in this regard war is obsolete. It's no longer needed. And then again, it's obsolete because nuclear weapons could destroy the whole universe. War, which once was controllable, could get out of control and so for these two reasons it's now obsolete.

TERRORISM – THE GREAT TOOL FOR "CONTROL"

There was a discussion of terrorism. Terrorism would be used widely in Europe and in other parts of the world. Terrorism at that time was thought would not be necessary in the United States. It could become necessary in the United States if the United States did not move rapidly enough into accepting the system. But at least in the foreseeable future it was not planned. And very benignly on their part. Maybe terrorism would not be required here, but the implication being that it would be indeed used if it was necessary.

Along with this came a bit of a scolding that Americans had had it too good anyway and just a little bit of terrorism would help convince Americans that the world is indeed a dangerous place or can be if we don't relinquish control to the proper authorities.

MONEY AND BANKING

There was discussion of money and banking. One statement was, "Inflation is infinite. You can put an infinite number of zeros after any number and put the decimals points wherever you want," as an indication that inflation is a TOOL of the controllers. Money would become predominantly credit. Money is primarily a credit thing, but exchange of money would be not cash or palpable things but electronic credit signals. People would carry money only in very small amounts for things like chewing gum and candy bars. Just pocket sorts of things. Any purchase of any significant amount would be done electronically. Earnings would be electronically entered into your Account.

It would be a single banking system. It may have the appearance of being more than one but ultimately and basically it would be one single banking system, so that when you got paid your pay would be entered for you into your account balance and then when you purchased anything at the point of purchase it would be deducted from your account balance and you would actually carry nothing with you.

Also computer records can be kept on whatever it was you purchased so that if you were purchasing too much of any particular item and some official wanted to know what you were doing with your money they could go back and review your purchases and determine what you were buying. There was a statement that any purchase of significant size like an automobile, bicycle, a refrigerator, a radio or television or whatever might have some sort of identification on it so it could be traced, so that very quickly anything which was either given away or stolen, whatever authorities would be able to establish who purchased it and when.

Computers would allow this to happen. The ability to save would be greatly curtailed. People would just not be able to save any considerable degree of wealth. There was some statement of recognition that wealth represents power, and wealth in the hands of a lot of people is not good for the people in charge, so if you save too much you might be taxed. The more you save the higher rate of tax on your savings so your savings really could never get very far. And also if you began to show a pattern of saving too much, you might have your pay cut. We would say, "Well, you're saving instead of spending. You really don't need all that money."

That basically the idea being to prevent people from accumulating any wealth which might have long-range disruptive influence on the system. People would be encouraged to use credit to borrow, and then also be encouraged to renege on their debt, so they would destroy their own credit. The idea here is that, again, if you're too stupid to handle credit wisely, this gives the authorities the opportunity to come down hard on you once you've shot your credit.

Electronic payments initially would all be based on different kinds of credit cards. These were already in use in 1969 to some extent. Not as much as now. But people would have credit cards with the electronic strip on it and once they got used to that then it would point out the advantage of having all of that combined into a single credit card, serving a single monetary system and then they won't have to carry around all that plastic.

So the next step would be the single card and then the next step would be to replace the single card with a skin implant. The single card could be lost or stolen, give rise to problems, could be exchanged with somebody else to confuse identity. The skin implant on the other hand would be not losable or counterfeitable or transferrable to another person so you and your accounts would be identified without any possibility of error. And the skin implants would have to be put some place that would be convenient to the skin, for example, your right hand or your forehead.

At that time when I heard this I was unfamiliar with the statements in the Book of Revelation. The speaker went on to say, "Now some of you people who read the Bible will attach significance to this to the Bible," but he went on to disclaim any biblical significance at all. This is just common sense of how the system could work and should work and there's no need to read any superstitious biblical principles into it. As I say, at the time I was not very familiar with the words of Revelations.

Shortly after, I became familiar with it and the significance of what he said really was striking. I'll never forget it.

BIG BROTHER IS WATCHING YOU, WHILE YOU'RE WATCHING TV

There was some mention, also, of implants that would lend themselves to surveillance by providing radio signals. This could be under the skin or a dental implant put in like a filling so that either fugitives or possibly other citizens could be identified by a certain frequency from his personal transmitter and could be located at any time or any place by any authority who wanted to find him. This would be particularly useful for somebody who broke out of prison.

There was more discussion of personal surveillance. One more thing was said, "You'll be watching television and somebody will be watching you at the same time at a central monitoring station." Television sets would have a device to enable this. The TV set would not have to be on in order for this to be operative. Also, the television set can be used to monitor what you are watching. People can tell what you're watching on TV and how you're reacting to what you're watching. And you would not know that you were being watched while you were watching your television.

How would we get people to accept these things into their homes? Well, people would buy them when they buy their own television. They won't know that they're there at first. This was described by what we now know as Cable TV to replace the antenna TV. When you buy a TV set this monitor would just be part of the set and most people would not have enough knowledge to know it was there in the beginning. And then the cable would be the means of carrying the surveillance message to the monitor. By the time people found out that this monitoring was going on, they would also be very dependent upon television for a number of things.

Just the way people are dependent upon the telephone today. One thing the television would be used for would-be purchases. You wouldn't have to leave your home to purchase. You just turn on your TV and there would be a way of interacting with your television channel to the store that you wanted to purchase. And you could flip the switch from place to place to choose a refrigerator or clothing. This would be both convenient, but it would also make you dependent on your television so the built-in monitor would be something you could not do without. There was some discussion of audio monitors, too, just in case the authorities wanted to hear what was going on in rooms other than where the television monitor was, and in regard to this the statement was made, "Any wire that went into your house, for example your telephone wire, could be used this way."

I remember this in particular because it was fairly near the end of the presentation and as we were leaving the meeting place, I said something to one of my colleagues about going home and pulling all of the wires out of my house, except I knew I couldn't get by without the telephone. And the colleague I spoke to just seemed numb. To this day, I don't think he even remembers what we talked about or what we heard that time, cause I've asked him. But at that time he seemed stunned.

Before all these changes would take place with electronic monitoring, it was mentioned that there would be service trucks all over the place, working on the wires and putting in new cables. This is how people who were on the inside would know how things were progressing.

PRIVATELY OWNED HOMES – "A THING OF THE PAST"

Privately owned housing would become a thing of the past. The cost of housing and financing housing would gradually be made so high that most people couldn't afford it. People who already owned their houses would be allowed to keep them but as years go by it would be more and more difficult for young people to buy a house. Young people would more and more become renters, particularly in apartments or condominiums. More and more unsold houses would stand vacant. People just couldn't buy them. But the cost of housing would not come down.

You'd right away think, well the vacant house, the price would come down, the people would buy it. But there was some statement to the effect that the price would be held high even though there were many available so that free market places would not operate. People would not be able to buy these and gradually more and more of the population would be forced into small apartments, small apartments which would not accommodate very many children. Then as the number of real homeowners diminished they would become a minority.

There would be no sympathy for them from the majority who dwelled in the apartments and then these homes could be taken by increased taxes or other regulations that would be detrimental to home ownership and would be acceptable to the majority. Ultimately, people would be assigned where they would live and it would be common to have nonfamily members living with you. This by way of your not knowing just how far you could trust anybody. This would all be under the control of a central housing authority. Have this in mind in 1990 when they ask, "How many bedrooms in your house? How many bathrooms in your house? Do you have a finished game room?"

This information is personal and is of no national interest to the government under our existing Constitution. But you'll be asked those questions and decide how you want to respond to them. When the new system takes over people will be expected to sign allegiance to it, indicating that they don't have any reservations or holding back to the old system. "There just won't be any room," he said, "for people who won't go along. We can't have such people cluttering up the place so such people would be taken to special places," And here I don't remember the exact words, but the inference I drew was that at these special places where they were taken, then they would not live very long. He may have said something like, "disposed of humanely," but I don't remember very precisely, just the impression the system was not going to support them when they would not go along with the system.

That would leave death as the only alternative. Somewhere in this vein he said there would not be any martyrs. When I first heard this I thought it meant the people would not be killed, but as the presentation developed what he meant was they would not be killed in such a way or disposed of in such a way that they could serve as inspiration to other people the way martyrs do. Rather he said something like this. "People will just disappear."

A FEW FINAL ITEMS …

Just a few additional items sort of thrown in here in the end which I failed to include where they belong more perfectly. First, the bringing in of the new system he said probably would occur on a weekend in the winter. Everything would shut down on Friday evening and Monday morning, when everybody wakened, there would be an announcement that the "New System" was in place. During the process of getting the United States ready for these changes everybody would be busier with less leisure time and less opportunity to really look about and see what was going on around them.

Also, there would be more changes and more difficulty in keeping up as far as one's investments. Investment instruments would be changing. Interest rates would be changing so that it would be a difficult job with keeping up with what you had already earned. Interesting about automobiles; it would look as though there were many varieties of automobiles, but when you look very closely there would be a great duplication. They would be made to look different with chrome and wheel covers and this sort of thing, but looking closely one would see that the same automobile was made by more than one manufacturer.

This recently was brought down to me when I was in a parking lot and saw a small Ford, I forgot the model, and a small Japanese automobile which were identical except for a number of things like the number of holes in the wheel cover and the chrome around the plate and the shape of the grill. But if you looked at the basic parts of the automobile, they were identical. They just happened to be parked side by side, where I was struck with this, and I was again reminded of what had been said many years ago.

The question then becomes what to do. I think first off, we must put our faith in God and pray and ask for his guidance. And secondly, do what we can to inform other individuals as much as possible, as much as they may be interested.

Unfortunately, some people just don't care, because they're preoccupied with getting along in their own personal endeavors. But, as much as possible, I think we should try to inform other people who may be interested. And again, put our faith and trust in God and pray constantly for his guidance and courage. To accept what we may be facing in the near future.

Rather than accept peace and justice which we hear so much now, it's a cliché. Let's insist on liberty and justice for all.

Source/Reference: US Coalition for Life, Box 315, Export, Penn 15632

CHAPTER 5

YOUR MORPHEUS MOMENT: THE SIMULATION FURTHER EXPOSED

"I am trying to free your mind, Neo. I can only show you the door. You're the one that has to walk through it."

– Morpheus speaking to Neo from *The Matrix* movie

This interview by Randy Engel, director of the US Coalition for Life, with Dr. Larry Dunegan, was taped on October 10, 1991, in Pittsburgh, Pennsylvania. On tapes one and two (made in 1988), Dr. Dunegan, spoke about his recollections of the lecture he attended in 1969 where Dr. Richard Day, an insider, revealed the plans for their New World System, aka the totalitarian, socialist World Government. Once again, this final tape/interview speaks for itself.

Randy Engel (**R.E.**): Why don't we open up with a little bit about the man who you are talking about on these tapes. Just a little profile and a little bit about his education and particularly his relationship with the population control establishment. I think that probably was his entry into much of this information.

Dr. Lawrence Dunegan, MD (**D.L.D.**): Yeah. Dr. Day was the chairman of the Department of Pediatrics at the University of Pittsburgh from about 1959 through '64, about that period of time, and then he left the University of Pittsburgh and went to fill the position of medical director of Planned Parenthood Federation of America.

R.E.: And that was what ... about 1965 to '68, about that period?

D.L.D.: About '64 or '65 till about '68 or '69, and then he left there. I don't know specifically why, I did not know him intimately. We were, you know, more than acquainted. I was a student and he would see me at lectures and, so he knew my name as a student, probably corrected some of my test scores and that sort of thing. Of course, I knew him as a lecturer would stand in front of the auditorium and listen as he talked about diseases and take notes.

R.E.: What's interesting is that this man is not as well-known, I think to our listeners as names like Mary Calderone and Alan Gootmacher. They were medical directors at one time or another for Planned Parenthood, but Dr. Day was not well-known. And as a matter of fact when I went back into the SIECUS archives there was very little information that had his actual name on it. So he was not one of the better known medical directors, but I'd say he probably had the scoop of what was going on as well, if not better, than any of the others before or after he came. Can you describe the scene of this particular lecture, the approximate date, and what was the occasion and then a little bit about the audience?

D.L.D.: The Pittsburgh Pediatric Society holds about four meetings each year where we have some speaker come in and talk about a medical topic related to pediatrics and this was our spring meeting. It's always late February or early part of March. This was in March, 1969, and it was held at a restaurant called the Lamont, which is well-known in Pittsburgh. Beautiful place. In attendance, I would say somewhere in the neighborhood of eighty people. Mostly physicians, if not exclusively physicians. Predominantly pediatricians, particularly pediatric surgeons and pediatric radiologists, other people who were involved in medical care of children, even though they might not be pediatricians as such.

R.E.: And the speech was given after the meal, I presume?

D.L.D.: A very nice meal and everyone was settled down, quite comfortable and quite filled and really in an ideal state to absorb what was coming.

R.E.: But when you listen to the tape, he says some of the most well not only outrageous things, but things you would think a pediatrician would kind of almost jump out of his seat at for example when he mentions the cancer cures. There were probably doctors in the audience who were perhaps treating a child or knowing of a child who was in need of a particular cancer cure. And to hear that some of these prescriptions for or treatments for cancer were sitting over at the Rockefeller Institute, and yet, as far as I got from the tape everyone just kind of sat there didn't say very much. I mean he was talking about falsifying scientific data and everyone just kind of yawns and how long did this speech go on?

D.L.D.: Two hours. He spoke for over two hours, which was longer than most of our speakers go and one of the interesting things he hasn't finished, it was getting late and he said, "There's much, much more, but we could be here all night but it's time to stop." And I think that's significant, that there was much more that we never heard. In the beginning of the presentation, I don't know whether I mentioned this at the introduction of the first tape or not, but somewhere in the beginning of this he said, "You will forget most or much of what I'm going to tell you tonight." And at the time I thought, well, sure, that's true. We tend to forget. You know, when somebody talks for hours you forget a lot of what they say. But, there is such a thing as the power of suggestion and I can't say for sure but I do wonder if this may not have been a suggestion when we were all full of a nice dinner and relaxed and listening we took that suggestion and forgot, because I know a number of my colleagues who were there when I would some years later say, "Do you remember when Dr. Day said this, or he said that or said the other?" They'd say, "Well, yeah, I kind of … is that what he said? You know I kind of remember that." But most were not very impressed, which to me was surprising because we'll use the example of cancer cures. But he said a number of things.

R.E.: Like doctors making too much money?

D.L.D.: Yeah, changing the image of the doctor. You're just going to be a high-paid technician rather than a professional who exercises independent judgment on behalf of his independent patient. A number of things that I thought should have been offensive and elicited a reaction from physicians because they were physicians. I was surprised at how little reaction there was to it. And then other things that I would have expected people to react to just because they were human beings and I think most of the people at the meeting subscribed more or less to the Judeo-Christian ethic and codes of behavior, and that was violated right and left. And particularly one of my friends I thought would be as disturbed as I was about this just sort of smiled wasn't disturbed at all. I thought, gee, this is surprising.

R.E.: Was part of it also because of his prominence? I mean he was.

D.L.D.: The authority, authority figure? Yeah, I think there might be something there. This is the authority. We sort of owe some deference here.

R.E.: And he couldn't possibly mean what he's saying or there couldn't possibly be any, I mean, he's such a good guy.

D.L.D.: I've often heard that phrase, "He's such a good guy. I can't believe he'd actually mean these things." I can only speculate about this. But I do think at the time there was an element of disbelief about all of this. Thinking, well this is somebody's fairy tale plan but it will never really happen because it's too outlandish. Of course we know step by step it is indeed happening right under our feet.

R.E.: Before talking about the specific areas, I think there's a lot of benefits from this tape. One of them is when we have a good idea of what the opposition is about and the techniques he's using, then you can turn around and begin your resistance to all the types of manipulations and so forth. So I think that seeing that there were four or five "theme songs" he kept repeating them over and over again. For example, this business which I think is so important that people fail to distinguish between the ostensible reason and the real reason. In other words, if you want someone to do something and you know that initially he'll be balky at doing that because it's against his morals or against his religious beliefs, you have to substitute another reason that will be acceptable. And then, after he accepts it and it's a faith accomplishment, then there's just no turning back.

D.L.D.: Right. It was in that connection that he said, "People don't ask the right questions." Too trusting. And this was directed, as I recall, mostly at Americans. I had the feeling he thought Europeans maybe were more skeptical and more sophisticated. That Americans are too trusting and don't ask the right questions.

R.E.: With regard to this almost a lack of discernment. I guess that's basically what he was saying. They were easily tricked or too trusting. The thing that flashed through my mind rather quickly, for example in schools how quickly so-called AIDS education was introduced. It did amaze me because if a group stated publicly that they wanted to introduce the concept of sodomy or initiate sex earlier and earlier in children and that was the reason given, most parents I presume wouldn't go for that. So you have to come up with another reason and of course the reason for this so-called AIDS education was to protect children from this disease. But actually, as it turns out, it's really been a great boon for the homosexual network, because through various things like "Project Ten" they now have access to our children from the youngest years. These programs are going on from K to 12 and I imagine well into college and beyond, so that they are reaching a tremendous segment. Speaking of children, I gather that this speaker kept on making the point about, well, old people, they're going to go by the wayside, so I presume that the emphasis for these controllers for this New World Order is really an emphasis on youth.

D.L.D.: Absolutely. Yes. Emphasis on youth. This was stated explicitly. People beyond a certain age they're set in their ways and you're not going to change them. They have values and they're going to stick to them. But you get to the youth when they're young, they're pliable. You mold them in the direction you want them to go. This is correct. They're targeting the young. They figure, "You old fogies that don't see it our way, you're going to be dying off or when the time comes we're going to get rid of you. But it's the youngsters we have to mold in the impression we want." Now something on homosexuality I want to expand on, I don't think this came out on the original tape, but there was, first of all, "We're going to promote homosexuality." And secondly "We recognize that it's bizarre abnormal behavior. But, this is another element in the law of the jungle, because people who are stupid enough to go along with this are not fit to inhabit the planet and they'll go by the wayside." I'm not stating this precisely the way he said it, but it wasn't too far from there where there was some mention of diseases being created. And when I remember the one statement and remember the other statement, I believe AIDS is a disease which has been created in the laboratory and I think that one purpose it serves is to get rid of people who are so stupid as to go along with our homosexual program. Let them wipe themselves out. Now it's hard for me to make clear how much of it I'm remembering with great confidence and how much is pure speculation. But as I synthesize this, this is I think what happens, "If you're dumb enough to be convinced by our promotion of homosexuality you don't deserve a place and you're going to fall by the wayside sooner or later. We'll be rid of you. We'll select out the people who will survive are those who are also smart enough not to be deluded by our propaganda." Does that make sense?

R.E.: Well, it certainly makes sense for them. And I think also this early sex initiation has the overall purpose, which I think we'll get to in depth a little later. But of the sexualization of the population when he said on the tape, basically, "Anything goes," I think that is what we're seeing. It's not so much that, let's say, someone may not adopt the homosexual style for himself, but as a result of the propaganda he certainly will be a lot more tolerant of that type of behavior too. So it's a desensitization, even for the individual who doesn't go over and accept it for himself.

D.L.D.: With the power of propaganda you dare not be against homosexuals, otherwise you get labeled homophobe.

You dare not be against any of our programs for women, otherwise you're a male chauvinist pig. It's like anti-Semitism. If this label gets enough currency in the culture that people get shockingly stuck with it. It's easier to keep quiet.

R.E.: Another theme was this business about "CHANGE." And I want to get to change in relation to religion and family, but during the period of hearing this tape, I remember going to a Mass and they happened to have at that point dancing girls from the altar. So when I was sitting and getting a chance to listen to the tape I thought, as a Catholic that has been if you talk about effective change, that has been probably the most difficult and the hardest thing has been to watch our traditional Mass, those things which Catholics have practiced and believed for so long and at about that time this speech was given, which was about late 1969, everything had begun to turn over on its head, so much so that I think many people feel now when they go into a church where there is the Novus Ordo, I think you're almost in a state of constant anxiety because you're not quite sure. What am I going to encounter now? You look at the little songbook; of course that's changed radically and you see, instead of brethren, you see people. Or you might see something odd happening up at the altar, which is now the "table." The notion of God as eternal and the teachings of Jesus Christ as eternal, and therefore the teachings of the church as eternal depends on the authority of God, and God brings about change in God's way. What this boils down to me is these people say, "No, we take the place of God; we establish what will change and what will not change, so if we say that homosexuality or anything is moral today, it wasn't yesterday, but it is today. We have said so, and therefore it's moral. We can change tomorrow. We can make it immoral again tomorrow." And this is the usurpation of the role of God to define what the peon, the ordinary person's supposed to believe.

D.L.D.: So, the idea is, that if everybody is used to change most people aren't going to ask, "Well who has decided what should be changed and how it should be changed"? Most people just go along with it, like hemlines, and shoe styles and that sort of thing. So it IS a usurpation of the rule of God, and if you read the *Humanist Manifesto*, and somewhere early in the introductory part of it, they say, "Human intellect is the highest good." Well, to any human being, what you call the highest good, that's your god. So to these people human intellect being the highest good is god. And where does human intellect reside? Well, in the brain of one or more human beings. So these people, in effect, I don't know think they'd be so candid as to say so, but whether they know it or not what they're saying is, "I am god. WE are gods, because we decide what is moral, what is moral tomorrow, what is going to be moral next year. WE determine change."

R.E.: That's right. And of course, in a nutshell, you've just explained the human potential, the New Age, all the new esoteric movements that we've seen. But with regard to change, he seemed to acknowledge that there were a couple of entities which traditionally blocked this change and therefore made people resistant to constant manipulation. And of course one of those is the family, and that would include grandmothers, grandfathers, our ethnic background and so forth and I guess I was impressed by everything he seemed to mention whether it was economics, music had the overall effect of diminishing the family and enhancing the power of the state. That was a constant theme, and therefore when we're evaluating things I think one of the things we should generally say to ourselves is, "What effect does that have on family life, and the family and I think if every congressman or senator asked that question we probably wouldn't have much action up on Capitol Hill, because almost everything coming down the pike has an effect of disavowing, hurting the family life and enhancing and expanding the power of government."

D.L.D.: It has an ostensible purpose, and then it has a REAL purpose.

R.E.: Yes, and as a so-called helping professional your ability to say that is very interesting. The other factor is this whole factor of religion, and he was talking basically about a religion without dogma, a religion that would have a little bit from all the other traditional religions so no one would really feel uncomfortable, and he said, rather condescending, some people need this and if they need it we'll manufacture something that they need. But of course it can't be anything that would declare anything that were moral absolutes or the natural law. Which means that the main target of this group of controllers of course, was and is the Roman Catholic Church and he mentioned the Roman Catholic Church specifically.

D.L.D.: Religion's important because it is eternal and we people who would follow the church will not buy our rules about change. But if we make our own religion, if we define what is religion then we can change it as it suits us. Yes, the Roman Catholic Church, I was kind of flattered sitting here as a catholic, hearing it pointed out that the church is the one obstacle that he said, "We have to change that. And once the Roman Catholic Church falls, the rest of Christianity will fall easily."

R.E.: I notice that, as the conversation went on, he said, "Now you may think Churches will stand in the way, but I want to tell you that they will HELP us," and he didn't say they will help us, all except the Roman Catholic Church he said, "They will help us," and unfortunately …

D.L.D.: He was right.

RE: He didn't say this explicitly, but again it was one of those themes that came through. He apparently thought the use of words was really important because he mentioned this with regard to a number of things, like the Bible. The very same psychiatrist, Miralu mentioned that "if you want to control the people, you control the language first." Words are weapons. He apparently knew that very well and I think the controllers as a whole know this very well. Of course, it's part of their campaign. But that little statement about words, that "words will be changed." When I heard that I thought, "Instead of saying 'altar' you say 'table.' Instead of saying 'sacrifice' you say 'meal' with regard to the Mass," and people say, "That's not important." Of course, you know that's very important, otherwise, why would they bother to change it? Otherwise, why go through all this rigmarole if it isn't important? It's obviously important for them because they know with the change of words you change ideas.

D.L.D.: They're exerting a lot of effort and time to change it and they're not exerting effort on things that are NOT important, so yes, you're absolutely right. The priest no longer has the role in some cases he no longer has the role the priest formerly had. Because words carry meaning. There's the dictionary definition, but I think we all know that certain words carry meaning that is a little bit hard to put into words, but they carry meaning. So yes, controlling the language you think in your language. You think to yourself in English or Spanish or whatever language you're familiar with, but when you think, you talk to yourself and you talk to yourself in words, just the way you talk to other people. And if you can control the language with which one person speaks to himself or one person speaks to another you've gone a long way towards controlling what that person is able, what he is capable of thinking, and that has both an inclusionary and an exclusionary component to it. You set the tone …

R.E.: Take the word "gay," for example. I have some old tapes by Franz Layhar and he talks about the gay Hussars, you know, the happy soldiers and now you couldn't quite use that same word, could you? But you know, the word homosexual, sodomite has been replaced with the term "gay," represents an ideology not only a word and when you use it, it's tacit to say, "Yes, I accept what your interpretation of this is."

D.L.D.: They probably had a committee working for months to pick which word they were going to use for this. The word "gay" carries a connotation, first of all, which is inaccurate. Most homosexuals are not at all gay. They tend to be pretty unhappy people. Despite all the publicity that tells them they can and should feel comfortable with what they're doing, most of them deep down inside don't.

R.E.: I suppose they're going to come up with a sad phobia for those who have a hang-up about sadomasochism and a pedophobia for those who have difficulties with pedophilia, so we can just look forward to this I think. I guess we can look forward to it to the extent we permit ourselves that we permit the opposition to have access to the brain.

D.L.D.: And to dictate the truth WE use. Sex education is NOT education. It's conditioning, and we should never use the term "sex education." It's a misnomer. If they control the vocabulary, then they can control the way we can think and the way we can express ideas among ourselves and to anybody. But "sex conditioning," "sex initiation" is much more accurate and we should insist on that. We should never use terms like "homophobia" and "gay." Homosexual is homosexual. It's not at all gay.

R.E.: That's right. In fact we're probably going to have to do some homework on probably all the popular movements in the US. Probably the pro-life movement is the most sensitive to words. Talking about media events and access to the brain, I remember the first speech Bush gave in, which he talked about the New World Order. I remember jumping halfway off my seat. That term. Here he is, the president, saying the New World Order as if it was something everyone knew about. And someone looking across the room said, "I heard that. What did he say"? And I said, "He said, 'New World Order'!" And they said, "What does that mean? Why is that extraordinary?" So, I think one of the weapons we have against the controllers is that if we can cut off his access to our mind then we have a shot at escaping the manipulation, if not totally—at least escape a portion of the manipulations. Remember, one of the books on Chinese POWs pointed out that some of their survivors in order NOT to be brainwashed broke their eardrums. And in that way, not being able to hear, the enemy could not have access to their brain and therefore they were able to survive where others did not. And in our popular culture we have a number of things, TV and radio probably primarily, that are the constant means by which the opposition has access to our brain and to our children's brains. So I think the logical conclusion, and one of the common-sense conclusions is that if you don't want the enemy to have access you have to cut off the lines of access which would be in homes to simply either eliminate altogether, or control by other forms.

D.L.D.: Take the networks at their word. They say, "If you don't like our programming, turn it off." And we should. We should say, "Yeah. You're right." And we should turn it off. And let the advertisers spend their money on an audience that isn't there. As a pediatrician I'm always interested in how kids do things and how kids are like adults, and whether you're talking about International politics where one nation goes to war with another or kids on the playground, there are certain things that are common. It's just that kids on the playgrounds do it on a smaller scale. But you mention cutting off access to your brain somebody says, I don't want to hear it. And I remember hearing kids on a playground somebody say, "Ya-na-na na naa-na," and they're teasing the kid. What's he doing? He puts his hands over his ears. Says I'm not going to listen. And the kid who's trying to torment him will try to pull his hands away and be sure that he listens. And it's the same.

R.E.: Words. Words entering. And the child knows. Words have meaning. They're hurting him.

D.L.D.: Goebels knew it. Lenin knew it. CBS knows it. It's interesting; the principle stands—across the board. It just gets more complicated as you get older. More sophisticated. But watch kids on a playground and you'll learn a whole lot about adults.

R.E.: Yes. We're all nodding our heads at that one. This Dr. Day was very much into the whole population control establishment, and he was of course in favor of abortion. But as he started talking about the aged and euthanasia I recall one of the population-control books saying that birth control without death control was meaningless. And one of the advantages in terms if one was favorable toward the killing of the aged, one of the favorable things is in fact abortion for the simple reason that, universally speaking, abortion has the result of bringing about a rather inordinate chopping off of population at the front end. That is, at the birth end. And the inevitable effect is that you will have a population that is top-heavy with a rapidly aging population, which is the current state in the United States. So, inevitably, if you are going to go about killing the young, especially at the pace we seem to have adapted ourselves to in this country, then invariably you're going to have to do something about all those aging populations. Because, the few children who are born, after all, they cannot be expected to carry this tremendous burden of all these people. So you're cutting one end and therefore, inevitably, as you pointed out on the tape, he was saying, "Well, these few young people who are permitted to be born will feel this inevitable burden on them and so they'll be more desensitized." They'll be more warmed up to the idea of grandma and grandpa having this little party and then shuffle them off to wherever they shuffle off to. And whether it's taking the "demise" pill or going to a death camp, or ...

D.L.D.: There was a movie out some time back called *Soylent Green*. Remember that movie? I didn't see the whole movie, but Edward G. Robinson liked to sit in the theater and listen to Beethoven's *Pastoral Symphony* as he was to take his death pill.

R.E.: That's right. He also made the point that the food the people were eating were each other. But as he said, as long as it's done with dignity and humanely like putting away your horse.

D.L.D.: That's a little bit like pornography. Years back kids would come across pornography. It was always poor photography and cheap paper. Then *Playboy* came out with the glossy pages and really good photography, so then pornography is no longer cheap. It's respectable. We went to a movie at the Pittsburgh Playhouse. I took my son along. It was the *Manchurian Candidate.* During the previews of the things that are going to come there was a title I don't remember but it was (inaudible) in Technicolor with classical music in the background. And it was a pornographic movie. And I said, well, if you have a guitar then it's pornography, but if you have classical movies then it converts it into art. It was pornography. It's an example of what you were saying. As long as it's done with dignity, that's what counts. If you kill someone with dignity, it's OK. If you have pornography with classical music it's art. That was the point I was trying to make.

R.E.: Again, talking about the family. Currently I know there are an awful lot of people who are out of jobs and he [Dr. Day] had quite a lot of things to say about, for example, heavy industry. I guess the shock was that of this man. I wasn't surprised that he knew a lot about population control, abortion, and at the other end, euthanasia. But what did surprise me was that he was an individual who was talking about religion, law, education, sports, entertainment, food. How could one individual have that much input? Now one could say, "Well, it didn't pan out." But we know listening to these recollections twenty years later, except perhaps for some minor things, everything that he has said has come to pass and almost beyond imagination. How could one individual talk with such authoritative, non-questioning that this was the way THIS was going to happen and THIS was going to happen in "fashion" and this was going to happen on TV and there were going to be video recorders before I ever heard of the word.

D.L.D.: I think what happens certainly one individual hears this, but the plans are by no means made by one or a small number of individuals. Just as industrial corporations which have a board of directors, with people from all sorts of activities who sit on the board of this corporation, and they say, "Now if we do this to our product, or if we expand in this area what will that do to banking? What will that do to clothing? What will that do, what impact, ripple effect will that have on other things?" And I'm sure that whoever makes these plans they have representatives from every area you can think of. So they'll have educators, they'll have clothing manufacturers—designers, architects across the board. I'm sure they get together and have meetings and plans and everybody puts in his input, just the way a military operation goes. What will the navy do? Will they bombard the shore? What will the air force do? Will they come in with air cover? What will the infantry do? It's the same thing. These people, when they plan, they don't miss a trick. They have experts in every field and they say, "Well, if we do this, that and the other John, what will that do to your operation?" And John will be in position to feed back, "Well this is what I think will happen." So it certainly covers a broad range of people. And for one individual to be able to say all of this in the two hours that he spoke to us, really tells us that he was privy to a lot of information.

R.E.: That's right. He must have been sitting in one of those boardrooms at least at some point. And I think not at the highest level from his position, but enough, because anyone in the population control would be associated with names of foundations, powerful foundations, powerful organizations.

D.L.D.: And I'm sure there was a lot in the plans that he never heard. He wasn't a four-star general in this outfit. He wouldn't be in on the whole story.

R.E.: Well, too bad he couldn't have talked for six hours instead of two, and we might have had a lot more information. There was another aspect that I found fascinating in listening to this. This whole aspect of privacy he mentioned that as the private homes went by we would have individuals, nonfamily members perhaps sharing our apartments. As I understand, that is becoming more popular in California. Could California and New York being coastal states, did he say, "That's right, port cities that bring in things so that they can eventually work their way to middle America." But this is about privacy. When he was talking, for example, about the area of sex, he made some interesting remarks. One of them that hit me like a ton of bricks was this business about, "We must be open about sex." As if there can't be any fear of the person that does not hesitate to open up to the public. Now, if you look at these so-called sex initiation programs in the schools where the children are forced either through writing or through verbal expression to talk about all aspects of the sexual sphere.

D.L.D.: Of our right to investigate even your sex life. Your money will be easy. We'll have it all on the computer.

We'll know more about it than you do. But we have to form a generation where the most intimate activity which two people can have is public, or can be public. Therefore, it's harder to have any private thoughts and you can't buck the system if everything you think and do is public knowledge. But the planners won't be that open about their own lives. They'll reserve their privacy. It's for the rest of us.

R.E.: Yes. Just like they're listening to concerts and operas, but for the mass media they're pumping in hard rock. That was another fascinating thing. For example, and I know this has come to pass because I deal with a lot of young people, the young people have their own radio stations for their music and adults have their own and never the twain shall meet. And when they do there's usually a clash. And I think the same is probably true with a lot of the classical movies. I can remember when I was growing up and my dad had the radio on, I think it was a kind of general music. I didn't say, "Dad, I don't like that music; turn to another station." Whereas now there is a fabricated generational gap which puts the family at the disadvantage.

D.L.D.: And it creates conflict within the family, which is one of the spin-off benefits to them. If you're constantly fussing at your kids, you don't like the music they're playing, and they're constantly fussing at you because they don't like what you're playing. That does bad things to the bonds of affection that you would like to be nurtured in the family.

R.E.: It would appear that any resistance movement against the population controllers would probably be based on families strengthening themselves in a number of ways. One of them being to make sure that children know about grandma and grandpa and where did they come from, getting out the family albums and making sure that children know they have roots, first of all. And secondly, that their family is stable. One father, one mother, with children, with grandfathers. Those of us who have them should hold on to them. Toward the end of the tape there was a reference at the time everything would be coming together—how this New World Order would be introduced to a population which, at this point I think they would assume would be acceptable to it how was this put? We're just going to wake up one morning and changes would just be there? What did he say about that?

D.L.D.: It was presented in what must be an oversimplified fashion, so with some qualifications, here's the recollections I have, that in the winter, and there was importance to the winter, on a weekend, like on a Friday an announcement would be made that this was or about to be in place. That the New World Order was now the system for the World and we all owe this New World Order our allegiance. And the reason for winter is that and this was stated people are less prone to travel in the winter, particularly if they live in an area where there's ice and snow. In summer it's easier to get up and go. And the reason for the weekend is, people who have questions about this, Saturday and Sunday everything's closed and they would not have an opportunity to raise questions, file a protest and say no. And just that period over the weekend would allow a desensitizing period so that when Monday came and people had an opportunity maybe to express some reservations about it, or even oppose it there would have been forty-eight hours to absorb the idea and get used to it.

R.E.: What about those who decided they didn't want to go along?

D.L.D.: Somewhere in there it was that because this is a "new authority" and it represents a change, then, from where your allegiance was presumed to be, people would be called on to publicly acknowledge their allegiance to the new authority. This would mean to sign an agreement or in some public way acknowledge that you accepted this authority. You accepted its legitimacy and there were two impressions I carried away. If you didn't and I'm not sure whether the two impressions are necessarily mutually exclusive because this wasn't explored in great detail one of them was that you would simply have nowhere to go. If you don't sign up then you can't get any electric impulses in your banking account and you won't have any electric impulses with which to pay your electric bill, or your mortgage or your food, and when your electric impulses are gone, then you have no means of livelihood.

R.E.: Could you get these things from other people, or would that be in other words, let's say if you had a sympathetic family.

D.L.D.: No you could not because the housing authority would keep close tabs on who is inhabiting any domicile. So the housing authority would be sure that everybody living there was authorized to live there.

R.E.: Could I get some food?

D.L.D.: Your expenditures, through electronic surveillance would be pretty tightly watched so if you were spending too much money at the supermarket, somebody would pick this up and say, "How come? What are you doing with all that food? You don't look that fat. You don't have that many people. We know you're not entertaining. What are you doing with all that food?" And these things then would alert the …

R.E.: I have seven people in my basement who object to the New World Order and I'm feeding them and then they said, well, one has to go.

D.L.D.: They don't belong there and you can't feed them and since you're sympathetic to them, maybe your allegiance isn't very trustworthy either.

R.E.: Yes. We see this, I think the Chinese experience tells us a great deal about certain things. For example, when they wanted to enforce the "One child family," they cut off all education for the second child. Your food rations were cut so you couldn't get the right amount of food, and if they found ways around that, they instituted compulsory abortions and compulsory plugging in of the IUDs. Somewhere in the tape this business is about "People can carry two conflicting ideas around or even espouse two conflicting ideas as long as they don't get too close together." And what immediately came to mind is here we have an organization like Planned Parenthood, "freedom to choose," yet they support population control programs, which is of course NOT the freedom to choose. And then when they're called into account and someone says, "Now wait a minute here. You're, 'freedom to choose—freedom to choose' here, but you're supporting the Chinese program, which is compulsory." I remember a statement from the late Alan Gootmacher, one of the medical directors of Planned Parenthood and he said, "Well, if people limit their families and do what we say, fine. But if we need compulsory population control, we're going to have it." What would happen with people who wouldn't go along, and particularly that point about, "There wouldn't be any martyrs"? That was significant, because I recall having watched some movies about the Third Reich that many times they would come late in the evening and people would be taken from their home, but neighbors would never ask, "Where did they go?" They knew where they went!

D.L.D.: Solzhenitsyn mentions that in *The Gulag Archipelago*.

R.E.: I think this is very similar to what we would see. People would just disappear and you would not ask because it might endanger yourself or your family. But you would know where they went. If you ask questions, you draw attention to yourself and then you might follow them to where they went. So you mind your own business and step over the starving man on the street who didn't go along.

D.L.D.: He didn't go into detail about precisely how this would come about but it's not too hard to imagine. Yes. In the past, the Nazis came, the communists came in the middle of the night, people just disappeared and one simple way to do this is that if you're cut off from all economic support and you have no place to live and nothing to eat, we already see a lot of homeless now. I just had a man in the office this morning talking about him and his child seeing people living in boxes in downtown Pittsburgh today. When the New World Order is here and you're living in a box, we can't have people littering the place, so you come around in the wagon and you pick them up. If your frame of mind as you're growing up and formed is that, "Human value resides in being productive; you have to have a prestigious position or at least perform something useful, make a contribution," and the truck comes by to pick up some guy living in a box and he's not making any contribution, who's going to get excited about it? You know, he's subhuman, he's a fetus, he's a zygote, he's a derelict, and fetuses and zygotes and derelicts are all the same animal. So what do you do with them? You dispose of them. Who gets excited about it?

R.E.: I recall that when the Chinese communists came into power one of the first things that they taught in schools was not any thoughts about specific political ideology, but about evolution and that man was just an animal and if man was just an animal then we won't mind being herded and having masters who keep tabs on the animals and we're one big ant colony and we've got someone to direct traffic and speaking of traffic. We talked about the aged and again, people hearing this tape, it's phenomenal how many times these things on this tape will hit you. I just came back from New Jersey, which has a lot of retirement-type villages, and I've been there over a period of years and there's a structure around a retirement home, which has been uncompleted for at least two or three years. Now they've recently completed it.

It's kind of a roadway, but I think it would be easier to get out of a complex at a playground. It is so complicated. And yet the whole area has elderly people driving. And we are a fairly middle-aged couple and for the life of me we couldn't figure out how we were going to get out, what we were going to do and so I asked some of the residents, "Doesn't it bother you that they haven't fixed this road for years and now you can't just go across the street, which would have been the logical thing?" You have to go down and they have a jughandle and you have to go over and under, so it takes you so long, and the woman replied to me, "Well you know, we just don't go out. We just don't go out." So here we have this little retirement village where they've made it very difficult for a population, maybe several hundred homes in this plot with only one exit and the exit involves such a great deal of bother, they say they just cut down on the number of times they have to go out shopping.

D.L.D.: Right away it makes me wonder if it's difficult to get out, it's also difficult to get in probably for visitors.

R.E.: These retirement homes sort of remind me of an elephant burial ground. The one thing you notice is that there are no children. There's not the laughter of children in these homes.

D.L.D.: My experience has been, these people in the retirement homes, when they see a child they just blossom. They're really delighted to see a child. Sure they're happy to have their sons and daughters come and other adults, but when they see a child and it doesn't have to be their own it has a very beneficial effect on their mood. And if these older people aren't seeing children, the other side of that coin is, the children aren't seeing older people either. So if you don't get used to seeing older people, they don't exist.

R.E.: And that's why, with the family, making sure your children see their grandparents very often, no matter how much that entails, the trouble with the logistics, etcetera ... it's certainly worthwhile because, again if you never see someone and you don't learn to love them and you never have any contact with them, when someone says, "Well it's time for your grandpa to check out," it's like, "Who's that?" Who's going to defend and fight for someone they never even saw before? Oh, I remember one of the phrases. So many of these things you only have to hear them once and they stick in your mind. It's so jarring. We've already discussed "sex without reproduction," then you also said the technology would be there for "reproduction without sex" and this is a whole other area because it's contradictory. If a land is so overpopulated, then you would want to diminish sexual activity, get rid of pornography, get rid of everything that was sexually stimulating. But, no. It's the contrary. You want to Increase sexual activity but only insofar as it doesn't lead to reproduction. That was the message, right?

D.L.D.: Yes, and this is my own extension. He didn't say this, but that leads to slavery because if you become enslaved to your gratification, whether it's sex, food or whatever, then you're more easily controlled, which is one of the reasons the celibate priesthood is so important. And so many priests don't even understand that. But if you're addicted to sex if sex is divorced from reproduction, something you do for gratification only, I won't try to parallel that with food because you can't go without food, then you can be more easily controlled by the availability or the removal of the availability of sex. So that can become an enslaving feature. Now, reproduction without sex what you would get then would have all the desirable attributes of a human being without any claim to human rights. The way we do it now, we say, you're human because you have a father and mother, you have a family and so you're a human being with human rights. But if your father was a petri dish and your mother was a test tube, how can you lay claim to human rights? You owe your existence to the laboratory, which conveys to you no human rights. And there is no God, so you can't go for any God-given human rights, so you're an ideal slave. You have all the attributes of a human being but you don't have any claim on rights.

R.E.: In *Brave New World* they had the caste system, the alphas, the omegas, etcetera. The way they brought about the different caste systems was that in the decanting, or birthing rooms, the individual who was to do menial or slave labor, work in the mines, received just a little bit of oxygen to the brain so they learned to love their slavery and they were very happy. They didn't know any better. They didn't have the wherewithal to do things, but the higher in the caste you got, the more oxygen you got to your brain. So we actually had a group of subhuman beings who loved their slavery. In the past slaves probably didn't love their slavery very much, but in this case, we have this technology which will make people love their slavery, and each caste loved being what they were in *Brave New World*. And any of our listeners who haven't read that recently.

D.L.D.: You may remember the slogan that was above the Nazi concentration camps something about, "Work is Peace and Work is Happiness." I don't remember if it was Buchenwald or Auschwitz. My recollection of words isn't precise, but the idea is what counts. And here's Huxley, writing *Brave New World*, saying basically the same thing before Hitler was even in power, so Huxley knew something.

R.E.: He came from a family that probably contributed at least in part to this New World Order. A number of the English authors, H. G. Wells from that period and from those associations who highlighted the concepts of what was coming down the path. I can remember reading *Brave New World* in high school, and thought, "Boy, is this fantasy land." Thirty years later I said, "This is scary." There seems to be a kind of a similarity between his writings and the talk given by Dr. Day, because you get kind of a mixed message in *Brave New World*, that these things are not really good. It would be better if man still had a sense of humor, a sense of privacy, if the family still existed … but, it's inevitable. They're going to go. Too bad. I feel a little sorry about that. A little sentiment, but the New Order has to come in and we have to make room for it. And I got that same impression from the things that were said about this Day tape. He wasn't really happy about some of the things, but they're going to occur anyway, so make it easier on yourself. The more you accept it the easier it's going to be when it comes around, and I'm kind of doing you a favor—you physicians out there this evening I'm going to make it easier for you by telling you in advance what's coming and you can make your own adjustments.

D.L.D.: Somewhere in Scripture, I think it was after the flood, God said, "I will write my law on man's hearts," and I feel the same parallel that you do between Dr. Day's reaction to what he was exposed to and mine seeming not totally accepting of this. Huxley seemed not totally accepting of what he wrote about but both saying, "Well, there's a certain inevitability to all of this, so let's try to talk about the best parts of it. It's going to be good for people. Technology will be better, quality of life will be better so you live a few years shorter." But they both do seem to send out messages not buying the whole package.

R.E.: And maybe wishing some people would ask more questions. Looking back over history there are many individuals who had an idea of what a New World Order should be, certainly Hitler and Stalin did, but what was lacking during these periods is that they lacked the technology to carry many of the things out, surveillance, constant monitoring, but in this so-called New World Order it's going to be very difficult to escape because technology will provide those means which had been lacking those totalitarian individuals from years ago.

D.L.D.: I can't remember on the original tapes, did I mention the phrase where he said, "This time we're going to do it right!"

R.E.: No. You didn't.

D.L.D.: There were so many details to remember. But when he mentioned bringing in the New World Order, he said, "This time we're going to do it right." And right away, I'm wondering, "What do you mean, 'this time'?" There was no explicit explanation of that, but I think it's fairly easy to infer that previous efforts had to do with the Third Reich. Your point about the technology is critical with computers and all means of exchange being controlled by electronic impulse. Nobody has any wealth. You own nothing of value except access to electronic impulses, which are beyond your control. A cashless society. So when your reward for working is nothing more than impulses on the computer and the only claim you have is these impulses and the people who run the system can give or take them as they choose. Up until this time there was no way the statement in the book of Revelation that said, "No man can buy or sell unless he has the mark of the beast," there's no way that could have been enforced. People could say I'll trade you a bushel of tomatoes for a bushel of wheat. If you'll drive my kids to school I'll give you six ears of corn. Bartering, and even not necessarily that primitive, there was always gold and silver and other forms of money that were even better than bartering. But with this cashless society, I believe this is the first time in the history of the human race where the entire population of the world can be controlled economically so that somebody can say, "I pushed the right buttons and I know how much credit you have electronically; I know where you spend your money electronically; and you cannot buy, you cannot sell unless you get on my computer."

Right now you have a half a dozen credit cards in your pocket, but pretty soon it will be narrowed to one credit card and then when we you know the ostensible reason is that when people lose their credit cards and we have to get rid of that and put the implant in where it has to be accessible to the scanner in your right hand or in your forehead.

R.E.: Speaking of scanner. When we had the TV war, the Gulf War? It was the first war where you just sit there and twenty-four hours a day just like being on the battlefield there. There were several points made about the advances in technology and how they could spot just one little individual down if they used the constant reference to "pinpoint." I imagine with the different technologies they can also pinpoint a couple of renegades in the New World Order. The technology which was applicable to a so-called "enemy" can also be applicable to this controlling the order.

D.R.D: Exactly. It's infrared stuff that's I'm sort of amateurish about this, but any heat source like a deer, a human being, a renegade can be picked up by an infrared scanner and you get sort of an outline of whether it's a deer or sheep or whatever. My first hearing about them was in the Vietnam War where our troops used them to detect the enemy. That's twenty-some years ago, so they're probably even more sophisticated now than they were then, but with this kind of surveillance it would be pretty hard for anybody to escape and say, "Well, I'm just going to go out into the mountains and be a hermit and escape the New World Order. I can shoot deer and eat berries and survive and I've got a wife who's pretty sturdy and she'll be able to survive and we'll do what the Indians did before Columbus got here and we'll all survive." The New World Order will say, "No you won't because we're gonna find you."

R.E.: Even in *Brave New World* they had a group of people who still lived as a family and the women breastfed and they were called savages. But we won't have any savages. We're cultured, we'll be thin and our teeth will be straight.

D.L.D.: Something also that was mentioned, forests could and if necessary would be leveled or burned. Now this comes out of this movement of goddess Mother Earth, and how we have to protect the environment, but if we want to get someone who's trying to get away we'll burn down the whole forest. We'll find them. That was stated. Deforestation could be and would be brought about to make sure that nobody gets outside the control of the system.

R.E.: We're drawing to a close here. How did you feel after, well, it's been about twenty-two years now since that original lecture and there probably isn't a day that goes by at least since I've heard the tape that I don't think about the things that Dr. Day said.

D.L.D.: You get constant reminders. Not a day goes by where something doesn't say, "That reminds me of ..." such and such, whether it's surveillance or security.

R.E.: Or clothing. I opened up a toy catalog the other day and noticed there didn't happen to be any baby dolls in this toy catalog, of course going back to the idea that we don't want little girls to think about babies. They only had one little doll and it was kind of an adult doll. And nothing that would raise anyone's maternal instincts. Well, Doc, what's the prognosis?

D.L.D.: Left to man alone I think the technology is already here and with technological progress, I think it is inevitable if man is left to his own devices that some men will be able to assert total control over other men, other people. Man left to his own devices the tendency is in groups like this, then is for internal dissension to arise where the leaders would be at each other's throats too each saying, "No, I'm more powerful than you. I deserve more than you."

R.E.: Who will control the controllers?

D.L.D.: Yeah. They would stab themselves. I think so. They would create their own seeds of destruction while they're creating the system. But the other thing I wonder if indeed this may be time for our Lord to come back and say, "Enough's enough. Because you're going to destroy my Planet Earth. I am in charge of the planet. I'm in charge of mankind. Mankind will be destroyed if I say. I will not allow my creatures to assume and exert this degree of control where you're going to destroy the whole thing."

R.E.: What I was just thinking as you were just saying that is that in the past, dictators could kill people, they could torture them, but essentially they could not change what it meant to be a human being. They could not change human nature. Now we are going to have this new "genome project," a multibillion-dollar project where they're going to be getting a tab on everyone's genes. No one shall escape. Everyone shall have their genetic codes and with this opens the door to manipulation to change the very meaning of what it means to be human. And if one has an entity then that no longer has free will, you just have to wonder if that point out Lord says, "Enough."

D.L.D.: Just as Lucifer set himself up as God in the beginning, some people now would set themselves up as God and say, "I control the computers, I control the genomes, I control everything, I am God," and at that point he would have to say, "No, you are not! I have to demonstrate to you, you're NOT. I'm still God. You're just a creature."

RE: And as you said on the original tape, we believe in what our Lord has said, in that He will not leave us orphans. He will be with us till the end of time.

D.L.D.: This right away now begs the questions, when they come around and say, "It's your turn to sign the allegiance form," what are you going to do? When Henry the Eighth came around and said, either sign here and join and while he was saying it they were throwing the noose over the limb of the oak tree, and slipping the noose around your neck and saying, "You want to sign this or do we slap the horse out from under you?" and a lot of people said I won't sign it and they were martyred. Despite his having said there will be no martyrs, certainly there will be martyrs. The implication of his statements were that they would not be recognized as martyrs, but there will be martyrs and they will be recognized as martyrs. Maybe not the same way as in the past but I think this is something people should sort of prepare themselves for. When I'm nose to nose with this choice, "Either sign this allegiance or we're going to put you in a boxcar and you're going out to Arizona, to the desert," I think we have to be prepared to make a decision.

R.E.: I think it would be an understatement to say that this tape has great meaning and it's like a forewarning and it gives us ideas of things we should do and things we shouldn't do and I think everybody listening to the tapes will come up with things he can do on a small scale. I think that's the beauty of this thing. As he was talking it wasn't real earth-shattering things he was talking about. He was talking about little things. Television. Things that we do every day. Things that are under our control. The books we read. And I think some of these changes if they are going to occur will occur with the individual person within that family, with him getting the word out and then doing the little things. I think they matter over the long haul, the most.

D.L.D.: Just as with the prisoners who survived the brainwashing, I think people who are spiritually oriented, who are thinking about God, thinking about their relationship with God, are the ones who will then be better prepared or equipped to survive this world and the next. Whereas, those who are just focused on meeting their needs right now, strictly the material needs of the day, they're more easily controlled. Under the threat of losing your comforts or losing your food or losing your head or whatever, certainly some people are going to yield, and those who I think will survive and I really mean both in this life and the next they're going to have to be the ones who are prepared because it's my belief when the time comes to make the decision. "Are you going to sign on or not?" It's too late to begin preparation and start saying, "Well, let me think about this." You won't have time to think about it. You're either going to say yes or no. I hope a lot of us make the right decision.

R.E.: I do so too, and I think the tape will change as many lives and have hopefully as good an effect as it had on mine and on yours and so let me thank you very much.

Source/Reference: US Coalition for Life, Box 315,
Export, Penn 15632

CHAPTER 6

THE ORACLE: KNOW THYSELF & THE SACRED SECRET

"You didn't come here to make a choice. You've already made it. You're here to try and understand why you made it."

– The Oracle speaking to Neo from *The Matrix* movie

Since the beginning of time, man has kept secrets. The most powerful of them were referred to as "sacred secrets." The most sacred of all secrets have been deliberately concealed from the public at large by the Medical Matrix. This was done purposefully so people would never truly know themselves or their true innate potential. The first step into "knowing thyself" is to understand the ancient esoteric "GOD concept" that exists within each and every person on this planet. Understanding this hidden concept puts the entire Medical Matrix simulation at great risk. This is why it has been kept out of the public domain and taught only to select individuals. The simulation could not risk that humanity ever discovers its innate G-O-D abilities. Generation (G) the ability to create life, Operation (O) the ability to support or sustain life and Dissolution (D) the ability to break down or destroy life. Collectively, these three abilities had been referred to as the "GOD concept within." The proper generational understanding and application of this concept would ultimately make the Medical Matrix obsolete. Thereby creating a great threat. The Rockefeller Foundation cannot allow humanity to discover this sacred secret that was imprinted within our DNA and expresses itself through the cosmic arrangement between man and his Creator. The simple fact you must understand is, man is not part of nature, rather man is nature.

To escape the Medical Matrix you must own the facts that health and healing come from within and not from any pill, potion or lotion. The following is your evidence. Cut your hand and observe what happens. Healing begins at the moment the injury occurs without your conscious thought or initiation. The body immediately goes into generation and operation modes innately and the injury heals by itself in time. Now, cut a dead body. Observe how it responds. Put every pill, potion and lotion on it. What happens? Nothing! Ask yourself why nothing? What is missing within a dead body and is present within a live person? Yes, the "generative" force of life, that is, dielectricity. Life is light and light is electricity, which creates thermogenic heat within the body to sustain its existence. Once the light is extinguished, so is life. The fact that the body moves is evidence of the presence and expression of force, motion, inertia and acceleration of dielectricity. When a person is capable of expressing more light through their nervous system, they have a greater ability to adapt to an ever-changing internal and external environment accordingly. That results in a stronger "adaptability factor" and optimal physical, chemical and mental health.

The secrets that threaten the Medical Matrix stronghold most are that of health, healing, vitality, longevity and physiological regeneration. Those who possess this ancient knowledge have the ability to control, manipulate and enslave the masses without them knowing it. Since 1913, Americans have become slaves to the Rockefeller Medical Matrix from birth until death. As a result, the sick are easy to control because they are dependent on a system they believe cares about them and was designed to cure their ailments. The Medical Matrix quickly and seamlessly becomes their master and they become its slaves. Sick people are also easily manipulated, because they are desperate and fearful. They see nothing but suffering, limitation and death in their future. As the Medical Matrix simulation daily runs through their mind, they become too afraid of dying and also unable to enjoy life. Most plugged in since birth, they blindly and faithfully follow those who control them. Medical doctors as agents of the system continue to fill patients' minds with fear, doubt and disbelief.

On the other hand, truth seekers who hold the knowledge and wisdom of the innate GOD concept and possess the sacred secret of physiological regeneration are "free" and become the "masters" of their own destiny. As George Gurdjieff articulates: "The first reason for man's inner slavery is his ignorance, and above all, his ignorance of himself. Without self-knowledge, without understanding the working and function of his machine, man cannot be free, he cannot govern himself and he will always remain a slave, and the plaything of the forces acting upon him. This is why in all ancient teachings the first demand at the beginning of the way to liberation was: 'Know Thyself.'"

All the priests of the ancient world were anatomists. They recognized and understood the fact that all the functions of nature were reproduced in miniature form within the human body. As a result, they used man as a textbook, teaching their initiates that to understand man was to understand the universe. These priests believed that every star in the sky, every element in the earth, and every function in nature was represented by a corresponding center, pole or activity within the human body.

The functions of the human body, the attributes of the human mind and the qualities of the human soul have been kept secret, hidden and protected by those of the ancient world through mythology, allegory and parable. The relationship between the ancient wisdom, the priesthood and the demigods was guarded and concealed for generations and only shared with those found to be worthy. For example, the Egyptian demigod Hermes brought forth to the human race the concept of "As above, so below. As within, so without." The religions of the past were all based on nature worship. They understood the fact that the human race was not part of nature, but rather an expression of nature itself. The priesthood taught its members what they truly are and how they could bring forth their innate powers that were rooted within the elements of life.

Such teachings empowered members to understand and remember that they are air. They were encouraged to breathe, observe, focus and decide how to take control of their lives. Next they were taught to understand and remember that they are fire. They were encouraged to burn, tame, adapt and ignite their inner power and potential. Thirdly, they were taught to understand and remember that they are water. They were encouraged to cry, cleanse, flow and let go of anything that wasn't helpful or constructive in their lives. Fourth, they were taught to understand and remember that they are earth. They were encouraged to build, give, ground and heal, as these were the foundations of a strong and solid life that would easily be passed down to generations that follow. Lastly, they were taught to understand and remember that they are spirit. They were encouraged to listen, know, connect and be still. This wisdom defined the meaning of life and empowered those who were worthy to have learned it.

These days unfortunately, everything within the Medical Matrix is about money, power and control. From birth, the Medical Matrix deliberately disconnects us from nature and as a result the human race as a whole suffers physically, chemically and mentally. It doesn't have to be this way. The future is what we make of it. It begins with asking, it grows with understanding and it changes with action. The power will once again be returned to humanity and to those who want and are willing to fight for it. The time is now to once again rebel and choose the "red pill" representing truth, freedom, knowledge, liberty and self-responsibility. Understanding that the Medical Matrix reality as we perceive it is false and that our leaders and institutions have deliberately been lying to us and have oppressed us to keep us weak. We must wake up and initiate our own "Red Pill Rebellion."

The choice is always yours, go "red pill" and don't be a customer or take the "blue pill," which represents the lie, conformity, the continued Medical Matrix illusion, worshiping at the altar of the white coat, blissful ignorance, believing whatever you want to believe while staying trapped within a medical system with no hope or desire to escape it. Whichever you choose the consequences are your responsibility and yours alone. You've always possessed the power to disconnect, but you had to learn it for yourself. You may have been born into the Medical Matrix against your will, but you don't have to remain there. You discovering this innate ability is what the Medical Matrix fears most.

CHAPTER 7

YOU ARE THE ONE: IT HAS ALWAYS BEEN ABOUT YOU!

"What is real? How do you define real? If real is what you can feel, smell, taste and see, then real is simply electrical signals interpreted by your brain. Don't think you are. Know you are. You have to let it all go, Neo. Fear, doubt, disbelief. FREE YOUR MIND!"

– Morpheus speaking to Neo from *The Matrix* movie

"Sooner or later you're going to realize, just as I did, there is a difference between knowing the path and walking the path."

– Morpheus speaking to Neo from *The Matrix* movie

You have been the "ONE" since the moment of your creation, but you have remained asleep since birth because the Medical Matrix wanted it that way. They fear your awakening because once you learn that you were born to be free, but raised to be a slave within their system, that knowledge is a direct threat to their control system. Once you understand the power that is encoded within your DNA that allows you to create life, maintain it and ultimately extinguish it, there is no turning back. I referred to this in the previous chapter as the "GOD concept" within man. G stands for Generation, O stands for Operation and D stands for Dissolution. This innate power within all of mankind, makes each and every person unfit to be a slave within any system. Your body represents the temple of the ever-living GOD. That is why as children many of us were taught that the area on the side of our head between our eye and ear was called the temple. The human body was created to be self-healing and self-regulating. It obeys only the laws of nature, in harmony with the sun, moon, earth and stars and nothing artificial. The universal dielectric power of the generative force that leads to your creation is also the same force that dictates your health, vitality and longevity. Sadly, you have never been made aware of this until now because the Medical Matrix was designed to create and maintain a steady flow of customers from life till death. The simulation even put into US law that, "Only a drug can treat, prevent or cure disease." If that was a fact and benefited the masses, then shouldn't the people on the most drugs be the healthiest? The fact that they are the sickest proves that we are definitely all stuck within a Medical Matrix simulation. Health, the way they promote it is simply an illusion projected to the masses, supported by their pills, potions and lotions to ensure the masses remain asleep, never challenge the system and remain docile and subservient from birth until death.

From today on, those days are over. Are you ready to walk the path? The time to wake up and embrace your true abilities and potential is now! Just because you were born into the Medical Matrix doesn't mean you have to remain within it. If you made it this far, you have chosen to take the "red pill" and have volunteered to become part of the Red Pill Rebellion. Waking up is not easy. For many it's terrifying because their beliefs are challenged. Others discover that their perceptions of reality can no longer be trusted. Many no longer feel secure because their truths, illusions and perceptions are destroyed. The most difficult part of all is to start over by unlearning and then relearning everything you were taught about medical doctors, the health care system, how your body works and what its true innate potential really is. Knowing this is not enough. You must do it. Those who truly become free take the difficult and necessary action steps required to bring about the change they so desperately seek. As a result, they will finally unplug from the Medical Matrix's sickness, slavery and obedience mindset installed within them from birth, throughout childhood and until death.

"Freedom isn't free. It requires rebellion." "There is no power without compliance." These statements were shared with you at the beginning of this book. I hope now they hold more truth, understanding and importance than earlier. You now understand that the Medical Matrix is your enemy because it has nothing to do with health and healing. It has everything to do with money, power and control. The Medical Matrix program was initiated to enslave you and your loved ones without your knowledge or consent. With its continued rapid expansion and collaboration with the government since 1913, you now have the evidence within this book of the first Great Reset conspiracy perpetrated against the people of the United States of America back in 1969.

Now it's 2024 and we all experienced the Medical Matrix's 2020 Great COVID experiment. They killed people, divided a country, broke up families and friendships, destroyed business, blamed some unknown origin, but yet the elite prospered, didn't play by the same rules, ignored the protocols and big corporations made more money than ever before. How was that possible? Well, the hidden hand of power used the same tactics as back in 1969, but this time on a large and global scale. Governments once again collaborated with the Medical Matrix to bring forth a program simulation that would further enslave the minds of people with the perceived false promises of safety and security for all. All that stood in the way of their complete global domination was the acceptance and compliance of the people. Those who remained plugged in or chose to take the "blue pill" bent the knee and blindly complied and did exactly as they were told. Others who chose the "red pill" were able to see through the lies, questioned everything and never complied with any form of tyranny that was presented before them. To all those brave men and women, "I salute you."

The government in collaboration with the Medical Matrix aggressively fed the public the "blue pill" over a four-year period of time and it played out as follows, "Two weeks to flatten the curve," "trust the science," "safe and effective," "wear a mask," "stay six feet apart," "take the shot so you don't give or spread COVID," "essential versus nonessential businesses and workers." Those who chose to take the "blue pill" did not resist, they gladly bent the knee and blindly trusted the government and its narrative. They willfully gave up their freedom and liberty for the illusion of safety and security.

Those of us who refused to drink the "Blue Corona Kool Aid," never bent the knee, we learned from our history and understood the government is not your friend and to never trust it or any Medical Matrix establishment. No time in history did either entity ever truly care about the health and well-being of the public at large. As the four years of the psyops continued, we kept our minds open, questioned everything, did our own research and acted accordingly using common sense, logic and reason. As a result, we remained free, healthy, strong-willed, defiant and emerged as the resistance within the "Red Pill Rebellion."

You are the ONE. It's always been about you. You are the medicine! What the Medical Matrix fears most is you waking up to this truth, understanding it and applying it within your daily life. They feed you fear and ignorance. You must embrace hope and knowledge. They want you to comply. You must remain defiant because without your compliance they have no power over you. They want you sick and push shots, potions and pills because sick people are docile, easy to manipulate and control. You must understand since you are the medicine, health and healing come from within, not from without. You must learn how to nurture nature because you are it, not part of it. Your objective must be to achieve an optimal level of physical, chemical and mental health and strength, while never bending the knee to tyranny of any kind. You must unplug and see through the lies. They want you to hate because that emotion drives division among all people and keeps the collective weak. You must learn to love and become the light that brings hope and people together because there is always less fear and more strength in numbers. You must understand that it is not what happens to you that determines your outcome, rather how you choose to respond. Choose NOT to be a customer of the Medical Matrix!

Choice expresses free will and always comes with consequences and repercussions. "Red pill" or "blue pill"? Either way, the Rockefeller Foundation's Medical Matrix simulation has and always will be a war for your mind, body and soul. By reading this book, you have chosen the "red pill" of truth, freedom and knowledge. As the ONE, you have to understand and apply the life-enhancing personal power of the following two facts: "Freedom isn't free. It requires rebellion" and "There is no power without compliance." The only true way to escape the Medical Matrix is through noncompliance and rebellion. As I stated at the very beginning of this book, "In a sick society, prioritizing one's health becomes the ultimate form of rebellion." Do NOT be a customer of the Rockefeller Foundation cartel. If you made it this far, consider yourself armed with the necessary knowledge. Embrace your deep, burning desire to finally be free and take the necessary action steps needed to protect yourself and those you love from the lies, corruption and tyranny of the Medical Matrix ... Welcome to the rebellion! Now go out and WIN!

ABOUT THE AUTHOR

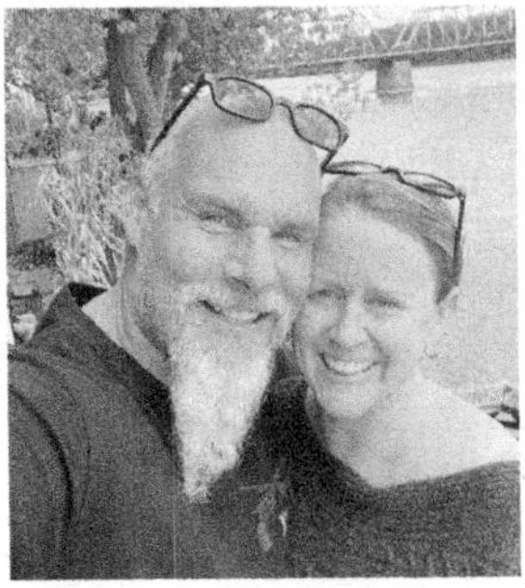

Dr. Vic Naumov, DC, a passionate, outspoken advocate for health care freedom, personal liberty and individual prosperity initiated his own personal "Red Pill Rebellion" in 1996 and won. In 2016, he wrote the explosive and groundbreaking book *Generation SICK: The Power, Politics and Propaganda Behind America's Health Crisis.* His book pulled the curtain and exposed the tyrannical truth about John D. Rockefeller Sr. and the "Medical Matrix" he orchestrated in 1913.

Married for thirty years, father of two adult sons, and soon-to-be grandfather, he and his wife, Colleen, successfully raised their children outside of the Medical Matrix becoming inspirational leaders and setting an example for other families to follow.

For over twenty-five years, Dr. Vic has been the owner of Naumov Health, a chiropractic and life-enhancement center, focused on not only treating, but more importantly teaching his practice members how they too can successfully unplug from the Medical Matrix. His purpose is to help clients amplify their innate potential physically, chemically and mentally. Dr. Vic currently lives in New Jersey with his family. Learn more at NaumovHealth.com and EscapeTheMedicalMatrix.com.